Advance Reviews for
Crisis Integration with
Acceptance and Commitment Therapy

"Much of my clinical work in addiction psychiatry focuses on engagement and acceptance: helping my patients, through motivational interviewing and mindfulness exercises, to engage the healthy parts of their neurobiology while tricking their brain to let go of cravings. This book brings it all together. It integrates masterfully the theory and practice of ACT and explains, step by step, how to work with a patient through the most seemingly-impossible-to-overcome crises."

Petros Levounis, M.D., M.A.

Professor and Chair, Department of Psychiatry, and Associate Dean for Professional Development, Rutgers New Jersey Medical School; Chief of Service, University Hospital; and Director, Northern New Jersey MAT Center of Excellence, Newark, New Jersey; President-Elect, American Psychiatric Association, Washington, DC; and co-author of *Motivational Interviewing for Clinical Practice*

"A guide to help clinicians manage and support patients in psychological crisis, this text is as warm and compassionate as it is scholarly and intellectually appealing. It firmly places mindfulness-based therapeutic strategies in the context of contemporary neuroscience and demonstrates their practical use with case vignettes that will move even a seasoned reader to tears. But it will also instill hope, by sketching out ways of adapting to adversity through inner change."

Markus Heilig, M.D., Ph.D.

Vice Chancellor's Professor of Psychiatry and Director, Center for Social and Affective Neuroscience, Linköping University, Linköping, Sweden; Member, Swedish Royal Academy of Sciences, Stockholm, Sweden; Fellow, American College of Neuropsychopharmacology, Brentwood, Tennessee; and author of *The Thirteenth Step: Addiction in the Age of Brain Science*

"Written in a highly accessible way by a world-class group of authors, this book shows how crisis integration can ensue from extremely challenging life experiences. It carefully walks the reader through the science and the theory and practice of how psychological flexibility may be acquired and taught. You will learn about each component of the flexibility processes and how they may alter the trajectory of people's lives. These processes apply to you and to the lives of those you serve. They apply to all of us. They are worth learning, and you have an excellent guide in front of you."

Steven C. Hayes, Ph.D.
Foundation Professor of Psychology, University of Nevada, Reno, Nevada; co-developer of acceptance and commitment therapy; and author of *A Liberated Mind*

"This is a masterful work on how to apply the wisdom of acceptance and commitment therapy to patients in crisis. Complex theory and research are covered in an easy-to-understand manner, but especially impressive are the concrete illustrations of how the concepts can be used with people who are suffering."

Kristin Neff, Ph.D.
Associate Professor, Department of Educational Psychology, University of Texas, Austin, Texas, and author of *Self-Compassion, Fierce Self-Compassion*, and *The Mindful Self-Compassion Workbook*

"We all experience a crisis at some point in our lives. And often our response makes things worse. This book shows us how the latest developments in psychology and neuroscience can help us to understand the nature of crisis and how best to respond. Metacognition, our ability to reflect on our thoughts and feelings, is the key."

Chris Frith, Ph.D.
Emeritus Professor of Neuropsychology, University College; Fellow, Royal Society and British Academy, London, United Kingdom; Fellow, American Association for the Advancement of Science, Washington, DC; and co-author of *What Makes Us Social?* and *Two Heads: Where Two Neuroscientists Explore How Our Brains Work Together With Other Brains*

"This is a beautiful book! It describes—with numerous explicit examples—patients in crisis and how we can help them to get through their crisis. Despite integrating the most recent and rather sophisticated science from psychology, psychiatry, and neuroscience, the book reads with a surprising ease and pleasant lightness. Intellectually quite challenging concepts are introduced without getting stuck in dry explanations and are well grounded in the phenomenology of body, mind, and life. This book is a must-read both for the experienced psychiatrist, because it bridges between clinical practice and the underlying theoretical concepts, and for the novice, because it teaches the practical tools needed to care for our patients."

Wolf Mehling, M.D., Ph.D.
Professor of Clinical Family and Community Medicine,
University of California, San Francisco, California

"*Crisis Integration With Acceptance and Commitment Therapy* is a well-researched, clearly organized practical guide for practitioners who wish to apply ACT to their work with patients experiencing crises. The authors delve into the nature of crisis and address its perceptual, somatic, emotional, conceptual, and behavioral dimensions in a comprehensive way. They build a conceptual framework for understanding how the elements of the ACT model foster resilience, and they offer ample practical techniques and clinical illustrations for working with crises and trauma. In addition, the neuroscience research supporting ACT's efficacy in terms of learning and behavior change is made explicit throughout. This book provides a superb balance between theory and practical applications."

Dan Clurman, M.A.
Professor of Psychology, Golden Gate University, San Francisco, California,
and co-author of *Let's Talk: An Essential Guide to Skillful Communication*

"Finally, we have what was really needed—a unification of the frameworks of cognitive neuroscience and psychiatric practice. This wonderful book provides real understanding of how the external environment influences the forming of the human mind."

Professor Martin Ingvar, M.D., Ph.D.
Barbro and Bernard Osher Professor of Integrative Medicine,
Karolinska Institutet, Stockholm, Sweden

"In the depths of crisis, we often find our greatest growth. *Crisis Integration With Acceptance and Commitment Therapy* is the guide that clinicians need to help their clients not just to overcome hardships but to emerge enriched in vitality and wisdom. A true delight!"

Poul Perris, M.D.
Psychotherapist and Director of the Swedish Institute for
CBT & Schema Therapy, Stockholm, Sweden

"The authors deliver a clear and heartfelt appreciation of mindfulness, with its different forms and uses, all solidly based on a rare combination of scientific understanding with deep personal practice. A hugely readable and informative volume."

Elizabeth English, Ph.D.

Teacher of Mindfulness, University of Cambridge, United Kingdom, and author of *Journeys to the Deep: A Gentle Guide to Mindfulness Meditation*

Crisis Integration
WITH Acceptance and Commitment Therapy

Theory and Practice

Crisis Integration
WITH Acceptance and Commitment Therapy

Theory and Practice

Katrina Carlsson, M.D., Ph.D.
Kirk D. Strosahl, Ph.D.
Laura Weiss Roberts, M.D., M.A.

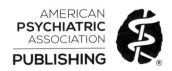
AMERICAN
PSYCHIATRIC
ASSOCIATION
PUBLISHING

If you wish to buy 50 or more copies of the same title, please go to www.appi.org/specialdiscounts for more information.

Copyright © 2024 American Psychiatric Association Publishing

ALL RIGHTS RESERVED

First Edition

Manufactured in the United States of America on acid-free paper
27 26 25 24 23   5 4 3 2 1

American Psychiatric Association Publishing
800 Maine Avenue SW, Suite 900
Washington, DC 20024-2812
www.appi.org

Library of Congress Cataloging-in-Publication Data
Names: Carlsson, Katrina, author. | Strosahl, Kirk, 1950- author. | Roberts, Laura
    Weiss, 1960- author. | American Psychiatric Association, issuing body.
Title: Crisis integration with acceptance and commitment therapy : theory and prac-
    tice / Katrina Carlsson, Kirk D. Strosahl, Laura Weiss Roberts.
Description: First edition. | Washington, D.C. : American Psychiatric Association Pub-
    lishing, [2024] | Includes bibliographical references and index.
Identifiers: LCCN 2023003915 (print) | LCCN 2023003916 (ebook) | ISBN 9781615373253
    (paperback) | ISBN 9781615374045 (ebook)
Subjects: MESH: Crisis Intervention | Psychological Distress | Acceptance and Com-
    mitment Therapy | Mindfulness
Classification: LCC RC489.C63 (print) | LCC RC489.C63 (ebook) | NLM WM 401 |
    DDC 616.89/1425—dc23/eng/20230320
LC record available at https://lccn.loc.gov/2023003915
LC ebook record available at https://lccn.loc.gov/2023003916

British Library Cataloguing in Publication Data
A CIP record is available from the British Library.

Contents

Introduction

*A*lthough crises may threaten to destroy us, they can also provide extraordinary opportunities for learning and growth. They are compelling and catalyzing as well as frightening and disheartening. Our goal in this book is to provide a new understanding of the dynamics of crisis—to make clear the psychological processes that can plunge people deeper into crisis and, conversely, bring them out of it. The skills that need to be developed to deescalate a crisis can also enhance the person's sense of vitality, ease, and purpose if they continue to use them after the crisis has passed. Thus, the abilities we describe in this book will be relevant to everyone's life.

We have written this book as a resource for psychiatrists and psychiatric residents, psychologists and psychotherapists, and other health care professionals who see patients in crisis, whether it be in an outpatient or inpatient clinic, an emergency room, a primary care office, or any other health care or social service setting. In all of these contexts, clinicians will be called upon to engage with patients undergoing crises ranging from acute and urgent life challenges to more chronic, multilayered sets of circumstances. Our aim has been to craft a clinical handbook that clearly describes the psychological skills patients will need in order to be with, deal with, and grow through crisis.

We have sought to offer clinicians a practical approach, underpinned by robust theory and evidence, to helping patients acquire these skills, often in time-limited conversations or a very limited number of visits. To this end, we present a simple, effective, yet counterintuitive way of understanding crises and what to do about them. Our approach uses a clinical model known as *acceptance and commitment therapy* (ACT) and a unique synergy of crisis science, evolutionary psychology, neuroscience, behavioral psychology, and the practice of mindfulness. These diverse fields all point in the same direction when it comes to comprehending what instigates a crisis and what can be done to help patients integrate crises in a healthy, life-enhancing way. Our premise is that, although crises can and do come in a great variety of forms, the underlying processes of the crisis response are basically the same.

This observation is hardly surprising. Having evolved through a long sequence of forebears, human beings perceive the world, learn about it, and coordinate responses to it in accordance with the ways the brain works. Our experience of the world—and of ourselves in it—comes as much, if not more, from the brain's guesses about it based on previous learning as it does from what is currently happening. What is experienced in the now is perceived through the lens of the past, just as our choices in the moment are to a large extent based on what has served us before. When there is a mismatch between the brain's guesses and what is actually going on, learning sometimes happens—but only sometimes. In the fear and agony of a crisis, we are particularly reluctant to update models of what previously—on both the personal and the evolutionary timeline—brought some degree of safety, relief, order, and care but now no longer does.

Fortunately, recent stages of evolution have bestowed upon the human brain an inherent ability to bear witness to whatever we experience, whether it be emotions, bodily sensations, thoughts, or impulses to action. Use of this higher-order ability can free us from subservience to our prior models of the world and generate the psychological flexibility that is needed in a crisis. Our capacity to observe allows us not only to experience the heartbreak of a crisis but also to recognize and to compassionately embrace our internal pain. We explore how such an attentive and accepting attitude toward inner turmoil will, paradoxically, reduce the sense of danger and burden commonly associated with emotional pain so we can better parse that pain for cues that will help us navigate the external quagmire of the crisis.

We have organized the book into two parts. Our aim in Part I is to introduce the ACT model of crisis instigation and crisis integration. In Chapter 1, "Crisis Fundamentals," we provide an overview of findings from the scientific study of crisis and of how the ACT model applies these findings in clinical practice. In Chapter 2, "The ACT Model of Crisis Instigation," we examine crisis responses from the perspective of evolution, neuroscience, and a behavioral-analytic account of human language and learning known as *relational frame theory*. Taken together, these approaches provide converging insights into the core processes underlying the generation and maintenance of a crisis. In Chapter 3, "The ACT Model of Crisis Integration," then, we show how the core ACT processes of mindfulness, acceptance, and engagement can be applied in clinical practice to healthily integrate a crisis.

In Part II we delve in depth into those three core processes. Our key argument is that when we stay present to our inner experiences, we are much more able to update our beliefs about ourselves and the world, to consider what we want for ourselves and for others, and to engage in actions geared to those aspirations. Here, mindfulness of the body is decisive. Building on the predictive coding theory of brain function, in Chapters 4 ("A Field Guide to Mindfulness") and 5 ("Mindfulness of Body and Feeling"), we explain how mindful attention to bodily states reduces our subjugation to prior models of our somatic and emotional states. This process sets the stage for greater acceptance of emotional pain and for beneficial new learning. In Chapter 6, "Acceptance and Self-Compassion," we uncover how self-compassion—bringing affection and kindness to ourselves during our most intense torment—can be crucial to acceptance and, conversely, how acceptance of distress enlarges our capacity for self-compassion. Finally, in Chapter 7 ("Engagement") we address another vital process in crisis integration: engagement with life. We can control neither what the world delivers us in the way of crisis-provoking events nor how we feel in response, but we *can* control our behavior. We can align the ways that we behave with the things that matter to us, even in the midst of tremendous distress. The ability to stay connected to, and be guided by, what we need and value—in the present moment and in our life as a whole—will give us a sense of purpose that enables us not just to survive amidst adversity but to thrive.

Because we have written this book for health care professionals, we demonstrate key principles through extensive use of clinical dialogues involving patients undergoing acute and chronic crises. Maurice (Chapter 3), for example, lost his partner and firstborn child during childbirth 2 weeks before his consultation. He stabilized his life for a few years, after having struggled with substance abuse and negative encounters with the law, but now he doesn't know how he can go on living. Another patient, Marina (Chapter 4), was found to be HIV-seropositive 7 years ago after a short relationship with a man who had failed to disclose his status. Her HIV condition is the first thing she thinks about when she wakes up and the last thing in her head before she goes to sleep. She loathes herself because of it and thinks about ending her life on an almost-daily basis. Lucía (Chapter 6) was emotionally and physically abused as a child by both her parents, and although she cares about her husband and two children, she has little trust in the world or in other people and struggles with long-term depression and suicidality. All of these case studies are based on real clinical practice and are presented in sufficient detail to illustrate how these and other patients, with the clinician's help, use their different experiences of crisis to discover purposeful new directions in their lives.

Katrina Carlsson, M.D., Ph.D.

Kirk D. Strosahl, Ph.D.

Laura Weiss Roberts, M.D., M.A.

Acknowledgments

*T*his book is the fruit of 25 years of seeking to understand the processes that will support people who are dealing with overwhelming hardship. It is the product of clinical work with patients, discussions with colleagues at the clinic of Norra Stockholms Psykiatri, and participation in brain research at the Karolinska Institute in Stockholm.

I am profoundly grateful to Anthony Nanson, my editor, whose guidance in the organization of the text was essential. His sharing of his expertise in the writing process sustained me throughout the writing of this book. He helped me to be more precise in my arguments and, since English is my second language, took on the delicate task of editing the text.

I greatly appreciate the generous and invaluable comments of Chris Frith on Chapter 5 and offer my sincere thanks to my friends and colleagues Ullvi Båve, Jenny White, Wolf Mehling, Max Kasun, Carl Gyllenhammar, Anna Mia Ekström, Eva Munk-Wikland, Sanna Due, Paula Blomquist, Judith Wolst, Chris Gilbert, Magnus Ekström, Cecilia Utas, and Johan Lundin Kleberg for their thoughtful insights. Any remaining errors in the book are of course our own. I would like to acknowledge a fruitful collaboration with Ullakarin Nyberg in creating ACT groups for suicidal patients, and my admiration of my patients, who have given me endless examples of how to be courageous and trusting in the most difficult circumstances. Many thanks also to Anna Björnström for stylish illustrations.

Heartfelt thanks to Marlys Mayfield for her inspiration over many years and for helping me shape the book proposal. My gratitude to my teachers of Insight Meditation, most especially Yanai Postelnik and Catherine McGee, runs very deep, as does my gratitude to Marshall Rosenberg, founder of Nonviolent Communication.

Special love and thanks to my husband, Torkel, for his unwavering support since the first bud of the idea of this book. Our daughter, Eira

Elise, is the delight of my life and I am forever grateful for how she keeps opening within me new dimensions of loving and learning.

Katrina Carlsson

*T*hanks beyond measure to my soul mate and life partner, Patti, for her seminal contributions to the development of ACT as a brief intervention and to the development of me as a spouse, parent, friend, clinician, and scholar. Thanks also to all of the clients I've worked with over the years who've demonstrated such amazing courage in their darkest moments. You've shown me what the human spirit can achieve by moving unflinchingly through the darkness within.

Kirk D. Strosahl

*W*ith gratitude to Katrina and Kirk and to Max. I have learned so much from each of you in preparing this lovely book.

Laura Weiss Roberts

Part I

THE FUNDAMENTALS

Crisis Fundamentals

We are here to love and to learn.

—Marlys Mayfield

Crisis and Learning

The idea that there's a connection between crisis and opportunities for learning is by no means new. Many stories in world culture deal creatively and primarily with crisis situations. A typical storyline in literature, theatre, or film involves a character facing an unexpected change that requires them to endure great hardships—often life-threatening ones—and to struggle to find the right response. Although there may be setbacks and failures along the way that deepen the crisis further, eventually the protagonist gains crucial insights that empower them to make a choice and constructively move forward in life.

For the audience or reader, it can be deeply satisfying to follow, and perhaps identify with, a character's journey through crisis—making mistakes, trying again, and, bit by bit, growing into a wiser, stronger, and broader human being. If the story is a tragedy, the protagonist may fail to learn some important lesson—one that may be learned by the audience even while they mourn the character's losses. If the story is a comedy, some achievement is recognized and celebrated by both protagonist and audience. Either way, such stories appeal to us in a deep and enduring way that suggests they carry some universal meaning.

The origins of Greek drama lay in religious ritual. Great drama provides a means of coming to terms with the fact that we don't have all the answers for all situations and enables us to learn from others how to embrace uncertainty and figure things out as we go. Drama is also a collective healing process that helps us accept that experiencing crisis provides a powerful impetus for growth. Even the word *crisis* comes from the Greek *krisis*—a vitally important and decisive state of things—which in turn originates from the Proto-Indo-European root *krei*, meaning to discriminate or distinguish (Harper 2020).

Nearly all of the world's great religions and philosophical traditions have likewise weighed in on the value of crisis. One important idea, going back thousands of years, is the transformative potential of facing a crisis. As the Sufi poet Rumi puts it: "Suffering is a gift. In it is hidden mercy." And the Buddha: "Pain is inevitable; suffering is optional." And the Bible: "We rejoice in our sufferings, knowing that suffering produces endurance, and endurance produces character and character produces hope." And the Talmud: "This too is for the good." And the Chinese philosopher Sun Tsu: "In the midst of chaos, there is also opportunity."

Whatever the wisdom of the ages, it appears that people today, from all manner of cultures and communities, are generally not well prepared to deal with crisis or even familiar with the idea that it is possible to strengthen one's capacity to deal with hardships, crisis, or full-blown catastrophe. Such skills are rarely taught in schools, in higher education, or even in the training of psychiatrists and psychologists. For the most part, we do not have access to any tools for dealing with stress beyond those modeled by our parents and peers as we were growing up or the strategies we found useful in dealing with the afflictions and shortcomings of our childhood context. Thus, we remain under-trained in how to relate and respond to a crisis or unable even to conceptualize what a crisis is in a useful way. Sometimes the very strategies we use will inflame the crisis, particularly when they are rigid and narrow—as they will be when they depend only on models and rules derived from previous learning. Whether the crisis is precipitated from change outside of us or by our own attitudes and behaviors, what is asked of us is flexibility—a radical flexibility implemented in tiny steps.

Crisis in Health Care Settings

When we fail to find a flexible response, when we have tried out every strategy we know and our efforts have failed to resolve the crisis, when our psychological distress has intensified, our mental health has deteriorated, or the crisis has metastasized into additional kinds of harm and further crises, then the time has come to reach out for professional help. Excluding scheduled follow-up and investigative appointments, the seeking of psychiatric support is in one way or another spurred by a downward spiral of increasing emotional distress that has reached crisis proportions. Therefore, crises are a common part of the picture in outpatient and hospital mental health care and indeed all health care settings.

The crises presented may be of high intensity or low intensity. They can be acute, bringing emotional urgency, or they can be prolonged and subdued, with layers of symptoms and complications accumulating over time. What determines the direction a crisis takes—toward growth or toward increasing difficulties—are the underlying processes. These processes must be addressed in order to understand the crisis and find the way through.

Dealing effectively with a clinical crisis requires the combined effort of both the patient and the psychiatrist. For the patient, it is a matter of becoming increasingly willing to face the painful emotions and bewilderment of unexpected and highly challenging circumstances and to try out new behavior in responding to the situation. For the psychiatrist, the challenge is to stay present and connected, to avoid falling into the trap of seeing the patient's emotional pain as an enemy to be vanquished, to access clear understanding of a crisis that presents in an opaque way, and to work with the patient to find creative pathways through confusion and complexity.

All these things may have to be undertaken while dealing with a patient who is distraught because of some catastrophic life change, is struggling to manage their sense of urgency, and is not necessarily willing to go along with the psychiatrist's game plan. Perhaps the greatest challenge for the psychiatrist in such situations is to keep a gentle yet steady hand on the tiller in order to respond with calm compassion for the patient (Roberts 2021).

The Benefit of a Functional Definition of Crisis

Everyone has a sense of what a crisis is. It is obvious to us when others are in a crisis. We intuit when we ourselves are in the middle of one—or at least know we have been in one as we look in the rearview mirror. The definition of *crisis*, however, is not carved in stone. There appear to be as many definitions as there are authors on the subject. Crises have previously been defined in terms of the type of change or stressful event that ignited them or the type of reaction that followed. Another widely held view of crisis is that it arises when life stress exceeds coping capacity in such a way as may lead to more danger (James and Gilliland 2012). In a nutshell, "a crisis is a crisis because the individual knows no response to deal with the situation" (Carkhuff and Berenson 1977), or we may say that a crisis is a person's experience of being overwhelmed and unable to deal with a situation by means of their present inner capacities and external resources.

Such definitions may be of little practical use to the psychiatrist trying to help the person in crisis. Yet if we accept the notion that the psychiatrist is not able simply to "fix" the patient's emotional pain or to eliminate the situation that is precipitating the crisis in the first place, these definitions of crisis do point toward the need to awaken and nurture the patient's own competences.

To learn more about which competences should be targeted, we must move from a *descriptive* definition of a crisis to a *functional* one. A crisis formula is needed that clearly specifies the functional processes that bring crisis into existence, so that the psychiatrist is in a position to reduce the influence of "crisis instigating" processes and increase the impact of "crisis integrating" processes. If the functional underpinnings of the crisis response are understood, the psychiatrist is already a step ahead in the search for creative responses to the situation.

ACT Model of Crisis Instigation

To the brute force of a major blow to their life, most people will experience an excruciating reaction—emotionally, somatically, perceptually, and conceptually. The question of whether this reaction develops into a crisis depends upon what one does next. A crisis emerges when an individual is confronted with an event, loss, or transition, however big or small, that requires them to respond in new ways, but, instead, they merely sustain patterns of previously learned perceptions, behavior, and strategies that are no longer helpful and may actually make things worse.

The functional definition of *crisis* that we present therefore comprises, first, a precipitating event and, second, an inflexible way of relating and responding to this challenge. Crisis doesn't come ready made; it arises from how people interact with change. From the ACT perspective, a crisis is instigated when someone does their best to avoid staying present to the internal effects triggered by life challenges and, at the same time, holds onto old behavioral strategies in response to an altered reality in which these no longer work. Crisis is defined here not as something solely imposed from the outside but rather as something arising from an internal response to an external event. We may be in pain or in a state of shock prompted by a difficult change, but that is not the same as crisis.

This definition is intended both to clarify the crisis situation of the individual and to point toward a feasible way out. The upside of a crisis is that it can excellently bring to our attention things we are doing that are not working and provide opportunities to investigate where our strategies for dealing with challenges are less than optimal. A crisis is not an aberration of nature; it is part and parcel of being alive.

No one should be blamed for unintentionally responding to change in a way that induces crisis. A therapeutic approach presupposes that everyone is doing the best they can with the cards they've been dealt. We are all acquainted with the humbling experience that, without guidance, it is nearly inevitable that we will continue doing what we have previously learned to do or will adopt strategies modeled by others. We also know that extreme and harsh events happen and that some underlying vulnerabilities are beyond our control. Not to be overlooked is the need for a social order that values providing safety and opportunities for all citizens.

ACT Model of Crisis Integration

In the Introduction to this book we mentioned the concept of psychological flexibility and the psychological processes that support it. The core principles of *acceptance* of what is going on inside and *engagement* in values-based living depend on an overarching capacity for *mindfulness*—that is, the ability to establish an observer perspective on and stay present to what is happening, both inside and outside. In practice, these three core processes of ACT are interwoven and enhance each other, so it does not matter whether we begin with one or another. In this book, we use the acronym ACT exclusively to refer to *acceptance and commitment therapy* (Hayes et al. 1999; Strosahl et al. 2012). Use of this acronym should not be confused with a three-step framework for crisis intervention—comprising "assessment, crisis intervention, and trauma treatment"—also known as ACT (Yeager and Roberts 2015).

Our task in a crisis is thus to learn to take advantage of our innate ability to lean out from our experience and observe ourselves with equanimity, curiosity, and kindness, and then lean again into the pain and develop responses consistent with our personal values. Clarity inside helps to shape appropriate responses outside. This novel task in a crisis contrasts with habits of doing whatever it takes to avoid what's going on in our emotions and our body, of not clarifying our values, and of letting rules and old reactions guide us through life's circumstances.

The key processes that are unhelpful and those that are helpful in a crisis stand at opposite ends of a continuum. The opposite of avoidance is acceptance. In this sense, acceptance has meaning only to the extent that avoidance is possible. Similarly, the opposite of being disconnected and numb is to be in the present moment and observant of one's responses, and the opposite of relying on old behavior and rules is to organize one's behavior around personal values. When we engage, we are involved in an ongoing process of contacting our present values and evaluating whether our strategies are consistent with those values. To engage means to recognize and apply whatever power we already possess. Engagement is a heartfelt, continuously chosen involvement in life.

Precipitating Events and Crisis Reactions

The ACT approach to crisis is process based and transdiagnostic. Thus it will apply to *any* crisis, preceded by *any* type of event, with *any* reaction, and with *any* underlying vulnerability or psychiatric condition. To affirm the distinctiveness of the ACT approach and to learn from previous research, we briefly review pertinent theories and results from the scientific study of crisis. Three ways that crises have previously been categorized are 1) by the type, intensity, and duration of the precipitating event; 2) by the type and intensity of symptoms and the duration of the after effects; and 3) by the scale—either communal or personal. Moreover, much interest has focused on individuals' underlying vulnerability to and resilience in crisis.

Typology of Precipitating Events

The kind of precipitating stressor that usually comes to mind when people talk about a life crisis involves an external event that happens out of the blue in a life that is otherwise proceeding quite steadily. A disrupting event drops into a reasonably benign life situation: something grabs your full attention, breaks the order, holds danger, has a drastic impact.

Many people with mental disorders find themselves with relatively few resources and may live in social environments already marked by continuous confrontation, danger, and conflict. In such fragile circumstances, a wide variety of changes—even small ones—can precipitate a crisis response. When little benevolence is available, it is easy to enter an almost continuous state of emotional distress. Even if we put aside these background factors, almost anything can precipitate a crisis if one responds to it in an inflexible way. Before we expand on what we mean by an inflexible way of relating and responding to change, we present a typology of life stressors that can bring on a crisis.

Traumatic Events

Although most people can handle such vicissitudes of life as serious illness, death of a loved one, or divorce, they may be overwhelmed by events that stand outside the usual range of human experience, such as "exposure to actual or threatened death, serious injury, or sexual violence" (American Psychiatric Association 2022). These are the kinds of events that have been formally defined, for diagnostic purposes, as "traumatic"—a category that also includes witnessing a traumatic event happening to someone else or hearing about a dear one experiencing such an event. The sad fact is that traumatic events are not exactly uncommon. Epidemiological surveys say that 80%–90% of us will face at least one traumatic event at some point in our life (Breslau 2009). Some of us will experience several over the course of our life.

Acute Events

Trauma is not the only stressor in town. Our locus of interest of this book encompasses minor and major changes and everything in between. Life's changes and stressors occupy a continuum—from low to mid to high—in intensity, duration, and proximity. They all bring challenges in their own way. Even a small stressor has the power to throw someone off balance in a way that may then snowball to produce greater impact further down the line if not attended to. Moreover, any change may have wider implications. The loss of a partner, for example, often also means a loss of external resources, such as income, knowledge, or a social network. Equally, loss of a job may mean a loss of income, colleagues, social context, and sense of direction. Sometimes we may face several independent changes simultaneously that, taken together, add up to major stress.

Chronic Stress

Acute events strike and then go, although they may have a long-lasting aftermath. Other unexpected events come to stay, such as health problems that become a chronic adverse life situation demanding extraordinary fortitude. There can be much complexity in the harmful situations endured over time by children raised in families in which there is abuse, addiction, or extreme poverty. The same goes for adults who are dealing with long-term unemployment or are trying to make ends meet at work or at home without adequate structural support. In such situations, a seemingly minor additional change can become the straw that breaks the proverbial camel's back—and so prompts the underlying complexity to surface.

Developmental Transitions and Existential Stress

We know that we must expect change as we grow up and grow older, yet the anticipation of transition from one developmental stage to another can be stressful. Transitions from childhood to adolescence, to young adulthood, to adulthood, to retirement and seniority, and to approaching death all bring challenges. Developmental crises arise when we fail to move on and master what life asks of us. Although crisis in response to life as it naturally unfolds may seem a more benign type of crisis, it is worth mentioning here because it helps to clarify reactions common in other crisis situations.

Existential stress has a different swing: unsettling agony regarding the meaning of life. One of the most charged existential turning points is getting ready to die—to leave our life and loved ones behind. The final separation.

Moral Distress and Moral Injury

Much of mental health is grounded in making choices in one's speech and behavior that accord with one's ethical values. However, to be human means to be imperfect. As much as we would like it to be otherwise, we sometimes find ourselves choosing and acting in ways that don't accord with our ethics—a misalignment that may induce moral distress. Whenever possible we can make amends and seek forgiveness—including from ourselves, which sometimes is the most difficult part. However, a common response is to avoid thinking about what we did that did not contribute to our or others' well-being, to put a lid on what happened, or to spend lots of energy justifying our actions while suppressing our distress, guilt, and bad conscience. The driving force sometimes is a misconceived fear that we will not survive if we admit having made a mistake. The effect of such avoidance is more long-term stress, sometimes carried over generations.

In the highly challenging setting of hospitals around the globe during the SARS-CoV-2 (COVID-19) pandemic, health care personnel were exposed to chronic stress because of inadequate resources, unimaginable workloads and long working hours; lack of contact with their children for weeks or even months; feelings of inadequacy and failure; depersonalized connection with patients while using protective equipment; and fear for their health and that of their patients and dear ones. They also experienced moral distress when they had to make difficult choices of prioritization in the face of human suffering that were sometimes not in accordance with their personal values and were based on insufficient information. This only added to their fatigue and conflicting emotions (Greenberg et al. 2020). In this kind of moral distress, you're doing the best you can in the circumstances, and yet you experience a dissonance between what you would like to do and what actually is possible.

Moral distress can also arise from witnessing or hearing about moral transgressions by others, as persistently happens in war situations, and can stem from the betrayal of one's core beliefs by a leader or a trusted authority (Griffin et al. 2019). In either case, such moral distress has been identified as contributing to emotional exhaustion, detachment, and disillusionment (Brenner et al. 2019; Coverdale et al. 2021). When moral distress is sustained or is related to a high-stakes situation, it may lead to longer-term psychological harm and impaired function—in other words, to moral injury (Griffin et al. 2019).

Major Disasters

Disasters strike quickly, and usually unexpectedly, and can cause tremendous harm, often to an extent that is difficult to imagine unless you have experienced it firsthand. Major disasters can be either natural or human-caused and can have both acute and long-term devastating effects, not only on individuals but also on families, communities, and the physical surroundings. Although disasters are not our major focus in this book, much can be learned from the development of humanitarian psychological first aid since the mid-twentieth century. Indeed, we should pay tribute to one such catastrophe: the Cocoanut Grove Fire of 1942 in Boston, Massachusetts, which was largely responsible for launching the scientific field of crisis theory.

As is often the case in personal catastrophes, larger-scale disasters tend to generate problems that extend beyond their immediate effects. During the COVID-19 pandemic, countries under economic strain postponed their attention to human rights and environmental protection and instead opened up for underregulated mining, for example, which in turn led to environmental strain and health problems among exposed populations. A disaster can even serve as an excuse to push through undemocratic and unethical decisions in favor of business or political interests. The initial disastrous event—a hurricane, a military conflict, a pandemic—is thus exacerbated by the chain of ensuing decisions that make things even worse for impoverished and disempowered populations (Kantamneni 2020; Klein 2008; Mustak 2022). In March 2020, the Secretary-General of the United Nations, António Guterres, called for a different itinerary in response to COVID-19: "Everything we do during and after this crisis must be with a strong focus on building more equal, inclusive and sustainable economies and societies that are more resilient in the face of pandemics, climate change, and the many other global challenges we face" (Guterres 2020). We see here two very different prospects of response to crises.

Perceptual, Somatic, Emotional, Conceptual, and Behavioral Crisis Reactions

Moving on from classifying crisis according to its precipitating event, we now explore what reactions to crisis may look like. It has been observed that crisis reactions have roughly two main phases. The first month is sometimes characterized by more acutely intense reactions (Bryant et al. 2011; Harvey and Bryant 2002). Thereafter, the person may enter a prolonged type of reaction with an enduring loss of psychological function and severe distress or proceed toward a healthy reorientation and integration of what has happened.

However rattling the experience of inner turmoil may be, a month is a relatively brief period. What happens next is crucial in determining the enduring effect on one's mental health and suffering. The field of crisis intervention theory has an entire research tradition attempting to answer the great questions we all ask: How prevalent is long-term psychopathology after stress? What generates and increases suffering during stress (taking a vulnerability-focused perspective)? Conversely, what protective mechanisms may shield us from developing enduring stress-related symptoms (taking a resilience-focused perspective)? In other words, why do some individuals facing a particular type of situation fall apart at the seams, while others facing exactly the same type of situation are able to grow in functional and spiritual stature? By looking at how the stressful event is approached and dealt with, the ACT model of crisis explains not only who will go in which direction but also *how* to promote personal growth—rather than collapse—in the midst of crisis.

Acute Crisis Reactions—the First Month

Acute and chaotic reactions are generally limited to the first month after a severely stressful event, loss, or major change or even after a seemingly minor change that nevertheless exceeds the person's present ability to accommodate it (Bryant et al. 2011; Harvey and Bryant 2002). Even when acute stress reactions don't take the most turbulent form, they can be a frightening experience, commonly producing a fear that they will last forever. It is good to know and to normalize for the patient that the intense chaos of the first month will wane with time.

Almost everybody is rattled immediately after an overwhelming change, suffering a disjunction of cognition, emotions, and behavior, as well as physical health problems. There are exceptions, of course; some retain their stability when encountering even severe stress. But painful and highly challenging change has the power to undermine the very basis of our understanding of life, our sense of meaning and purpose, our goals and role in the world, our way of living. What has happened seems unbelievable and illusory. Repetitive and intrusive thoughts and vivid images that appear for no apparent reason can also be part of the picture. Even those who seem composed from the outside may be experiencing chaos and confusion within. The disbelief and cognitive disorientation commonly obstruct one from taking in new information, both about the changed reality and in the form of advice from those who want to help. The new situation is fully integrated little by little and only with time.

During this first phase of a crisis, we may experience a continuous resurgence of intense and distressing emotions: fear, sadness, mourning, yearning, guilt, irritability, anger, or numbness. Stress hormones are circulating, mobilizing bodily reactions so that we experience a rapid heartbeat, sweating, tenseness, discomfort, gastric symptoms such as nausea and loose bowels, a headache, and sleep disturbances. Sleep problems are especially important to watch for because they increase vulnerability. It is common to lose both appetite and the ability to sleep well, although some individuals may overeat and oversleep. During stress, sensitivity to all types of sensory input is heightened; sounds, smells, and sights may feel exaggerated and obtrusive and, in some cases, activate the memory of the precipitating event. Images or memories relating to the event can also surface for seemingly no reason, with no volition, during the day or in dreams at night. Elevated arousal symptoms and hypervigilance may cause difficulty concentrating on the most basic tasks. Behavioral patterns can be disruptive or be characterized by inactivity and quiet. Conflict and frequent disagreements may be provoked that lead in turn to strained relationships, or the person may become withdrawn and seek isolation.

When someone is overwhelmed by crisis, moreover, it is not unusual to demand a quick fix. The intense emotion and the intrusive confused thoughts make us want a remedy. We may think that sustained contact with distressing and unwanted private experiences is dangerous or a sign of poor health and that to restore our health we need to control or eliminate these experiences by any means possible. However, crises tend to be complex, especially when they stem from longer-term problems, and so will only be resolved in ways that have yet to be learned. Major decisions made in an attempt to escape the situation or distress are therefore not appropriate during acute crisis; they only exacerbate the situation. Likewise, retreating into familiar habits—even when they are counterproductive in the changed situation—in an attempt to find stability may give the appearance of resolving the crisis, but this situation is precarious, especially when the behavioral and psychological mechanisms on which this apparent resolution depends are actually part of the problem. If you don't face the crisis directly, then you're retreating from what is actually happening; you're estranged from your own reality.

Periods of emotional and cognitive agony can often be interspersed with periods of ease, humor, and effective reasoning and problem-solving, which is a sign of a good prognosis. This pendulum between torment and ease can be made less confusing if one learns that this is a common experience. A persistently negative mood and an inability to experience positive emotions at all are warning signs that the person may be at risk of more lasting distress (Feder et al. 2016).

Prolonged Crisis Reactions—What Happens Next?

It goes without saying that we find heterogeneity in the lasting response to painful change. What is interesting, however, is that the variation in response to a challenging and stressful event manifests in a relatively small set of prototypical outcome trajectories. Some people are not affected at all by the negative event in terms of experiencing despair or anxiety, for example, or difficulty sleeping, working, or caring for their families. Some experience acute reactions but after about a month will return to stability in performing important functions. In Figure 1–1, such situations are labeled as *no/low symptom*. Others develop psychiatric symptoms accompanied by disruption of their ability to meet role obligations, but over time they *improve* and return to healthy functioning within a few years. The third trajectory involves the development of *chronic* suffering and the loss of important functions. The fourth and least common trajectory is a *delayed* display of symptoms that then worsen over time (see Figure 1–1) (Bonanno et al. 2011; Feder et al. 2016; Norris et al. 2009; Southwick et al. 2014).

How do we know we're dealing with a prolonged crisis reaction? Crisis research defines long-term outcomes according to the maxim "You have to draw the line somewhere," using the most unambiguous measurement of outcomes of psychopathology versus non-psychopathology. Among the general population who are exposed to trauma, typically 5%–10% (and up to one-third) develop PTSD. Up to 25% of those exposed to trauma develop major depressive disorder. Substance abuse problems may develop or preexisting problems may worsen or recur (North and Pfefferbaum 2013). Unsurprisingly, PTSD, depression, and substance abuse tend to co-occur. With traumas that result in grief, conditions such as prolonged grief disorder (PGD) may ensue (American Psychiatric Association 2022; Prigerson et al. 2021; Zisook and Shear 2009). Suicide risk increases after a negative

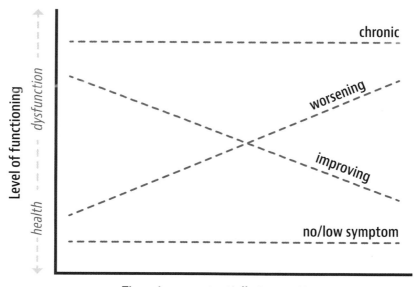

Figure 1–1.   Outcome trajectories after a potentially traumatic event.

Source.   Adapted from Bonanno et al. 2011; Feder et al. 2016.

life event (Gradus et al. 2010; Haglund et al. 2019), just as it does in response to long-term unresolved crises generated by early life adversity, such as parental neglect or childhood abuse (Turecki and Brent 2016).

Although crisis is widely and typically thought of as the expression of reactions during the first acute period of turbulence, the psychopathology that evolves afterward is an important part of the picture. In this book, we recognize crisis reactions of not only short but also long duration, sometimes lingering for years and years. Whether brief or prolonged, crisis responses can ultimately be life threatening. Moreover, our argument does not center on whether patients fulfill diagnostic criteria after a life catastrophe; it recognizes any significant levels of suffering and loss of function that relate to the "crisis." Finally, when patients have particular vulnerabilities, it is important to learn about any processes that are exacerbating their crisis and to access processes that will strengthen their capacity to move through challenges both great and small. Before taking a closer look at these processes, we must first look at what is meant by "vulnerability."

Vulnerability and Resilience

Intense research has sought to work out what will be set in motion after a stressful event—whether personal growth or longer-term dysfunction (Southwick and Charney 2012a). There's also a great deal of public interest in this issue. We can ask the question in terms of what factors contribute to vulnerability to disorder after the experience of stress, or, conversely, we can ask what facilitates the maintenance of mental health after someone has undergone severe physical or psychological challenges (Kalisch et al. 2017). High-quality knowledge has been gained from both clinical disorder–focused and mental health–focused research.

Vulnerability Factors Linked to Mental Health

There is no debate that psychiatric symptoms are connected to underlying vulnerabilities. From epidemiological and twin studies that measure the variation of mental health in the population, we can learn about biological, psychological, and sociological factors associated with psychiatric symptoms. There are genetic factors, for example (Lee et al. 2019). Epigenetic changes, which are often brought about during sensitive periods of development, regulate gene expression (Roth and Sweatt 2011). Susceptibility to poor mental health is associated with attachment style—the type of bond that is formed with one's primary caregiver early on and influences later relationships (Asch et al. 2021a; Bowlby 1980; Brumariu and Kerns 2010; Widom et al. 2018)—and with early trauma (Hailes et al. 2019). Thus, children who experience deprivation, neglect, or trauma early in life may have heightened vulnerability later in life. External factors such as social support, residential stability, and economic security are also known to influence mental health (Rohde et al. 2016; Southwick and Charney 2012b; Tol et al. 2011).

More than 40 years ago, long before such data were available, Zubin and Spring (1977) related stress and vulnerability in a model of how psychotic symptoms emerge (Figure 1–2). This model has been used frequently ever since, thanks to the simplicity with which it demonstrates how a seemingly minor stressor can elicit symptoms when an underlying vulnerability exists. A problem that one person can easily take in stride may be enough to cause another to become psychotic. At the other pole, the model illustrates how when vulnerability is trivial, extraordinary stress, such as the hellish conditions of trench warfare in World War I, can produce a common experience of psychotic symptoms. Almost anyone can become overwhelmed by a challenge of sufficient magnitude and duration (Carrión 2018; Hobfoll et al. 2011).

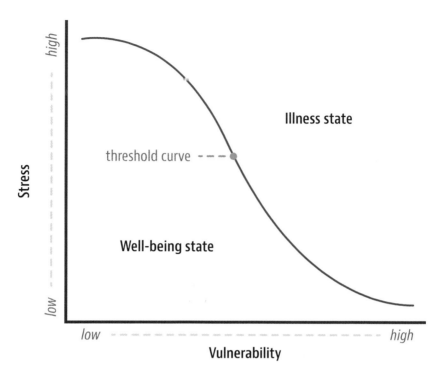

Figure 1–2.   Stress and vulnerability model.

Source.   Adapted from Zubin and Spring 1977.

Resilience Processes

Turning from questions of vulnerability to suffering in times of stress and attending instead to what contributes to resilience, we move from disorder-focused to health-focused research. Are there any traits and processes that will help us maintain good health and even develop abilities and new skills in response to adversities? Certainly, there must be some. For example, nearly 70% of war veterans, a population who will have endured a high number of harmful events, report minimal or no long-term psychological distress (Isaacs et al. 2017).

In scientific studies, *resilience* previously was defined as a set of *predisposing factors* that are more or less juxtaposed with vulnerability factors. Framed as something already present before a stressful event and relatively stable across time, it was typically described in terms of personality traits (Bonanno and Diminich 2013). Since the 1970s, this trait-oriented perspective has not only been the focus of science but has abounded in popular psychology and in everyday discourse and understanding. Lately, resilience has even become a buzzword of sorts, used in such a way as to suggest that certain fixed characteristics of an individual are protective during times of challenge.

Let us fast forward and lay out the cards. In studies of general populations, what has so far been found is that individual traits that existed before a challenge appear to account for very little of how resilient a person turns out to be. No property of personality has been found empirically to explain more than a few percent of outcome variance in the general population—or, in other words, to explain who will eventually end up with psychopathology and who will not after exposure to severe stress (Kalisch et al. 2017). There seems to be very little that is fixed or certain about how a particular person will respond to a particular type of crisis.

In the 80 years of research since the Cocoanut Grove fire, science has advanced to the point of proposing that resilience is an outcome from a dynamic process relating to the stressful event (Bonanno 2021a; Kalisch et al. 2017). This puts the notion of resilience exactly in line with the ACT approach to crisis as outlined earlier. Individuals change as they successfully respond to adversities; they alter their perspective on life, themselves, and others and gain new skills. The process of resilience is a complex time-varying interaction between the individual, the context, and the stressful event that arises during the stressful situation. When we are exposed to unfortunate events, *how* we integrate and respond to them determines whether a prolonged crisis will emerge—whether we will go into a downward spiral or grow and evolve through the event. Rather than something fixed, something that exists before, during, and after stress, resilience is the active process of relating and responding to stress (Bonanno 2021a; Kalisch et al. 2017).

There is no contradiction in framing resilience as a process and vulnerabilities as predisposing factors for mental illness. It's not a matter of "either/or" but rather of "both/and." Vulnerabilities to developing mental illnesses do exist, *and* there are both helpful and unhelpful processes in experiencing and dealing with challenges. To bring about real change, we must address both of these dimensions.

In clinical work, gaining greater understanding of the patient's state of mental health, together with use of an appropriate pharmacological choice, often marks an important turning point for people in crisis who display psychiatric symptoms. Sometimes, for example, when the pressure of a depression is eased, an impetus toward a fulfilling life awakens. Often, however, this is not the whole story of mental health; most of the time, the dynamic skills of living in harmony with life's challenges must be practiced alongside addressing any underlying vulnerability.

Those bearing vulnerability have an even greater need than others to develop competences for dealing with daily hassles and acute burdens in order to avoid further relapses into clinical symptoms and crisis—or for dealing with crises that do arise. It is a humbling experience to listen to and take in the immensity of stress, adversity, uncertainty with which patients are often grappling. Just getting themselves through each day often takes a heroic effort. Moreover, the initial phase of a mental disorder, such as a first psychotic episode, can itself lead to a crisis and hence a need for developing the appropriate tools to process this difficult new turn in life.

Finally, many factors contributing to vulnerability are unavailable to regulation in a crisis consultation, whereas dynamic resilience processes—things one can use in the present moment—will help empower the patient to change the trajectory of development, both internally and externally.

Research on Resilience and ACT

In studying resilience, we would ideally want to collect data—including health scores—before, during, and after exposure to the stressor. Such prospective studies are time and resource hungry, and presently rather few, but their number is increasing. Major stressors that affect large populations, such as the 9/11 terrorist attack, present opportunities to sample data from many individuals and to gather information about possible mitigators such as perceived social support or problem-solving skills. The prospective collection of outcome data will increase the quality of the study because it is easier to describe your present status than to accurately remember how things were in the past. Moreover, collecting the data at several time points enables us to learn about health trajectories and the factors influencing them. If these factors, such as social support, covary over time with a better outcome, the conclusion can be drawn that they probably decrease the risk of a prolonged crisis reaction. Important information can also be extracted from qualitative studies in which, for example, resilient people are interviewed (Southwick and Charney 2012b).

At the top of the hierarchy of knowledge about cause and effect in evidence-based medicine are randomized controlled trials (RCTs). These gold-standard studies involve experimental designs in which groups are assigned to different types of interventions or to no intervention. However, not only are RCTs on crisis difficult to do but, when the population in question consists of individuals who have just been exposed to acute and severe stress, there are also inherent ethical questions: how to obtain authentic informed consent for gathering data or implementing interventions from a person who is in the midst of a life crisis, or how to organize large-scale scientific trials in a major disaster setting where even the provision of basic needs and safety is a challenge. Even the psychological first aid outlined and recommended worldwide by the World Health Organization (WHO) for major disasters has not been thoroughly tested and should therefore be understood as evidence-informed rather than evidence-based (Fox et al. 2012; North and Pfefferbaum 2013).

Refugees of war experience prolonged and intense stress, sometimes for years on end, and have a high risk of developing conditions such as PTSD and depression. Two recent RCTs examining the effectiveness of ACT have been performed in adverse settings of this long-term kind. One trial, performed with Syrian refugees in Turkey, became the first *preventive* RCT to provide evidence that refugees of war receiving a psychological intervention were less likely to develop a psychiatric condition: participants in the ACT group were significantly less likely to have any psychiatric condition at 6-month follow-up than those in the control group (22% vs. 41%) (Acarturk et al. 2022). In an RCT performed in Uganda with South Sudanese refugees, participants were already experiencing considerable psychological distress, including PTSD and depression. Those who received an ACT self-help intervention demonstrated stronger improvement after 3 months than those in the control group (Tol et al. 2020). The psychological intervention in both of these studies was delivered by facilitators who had no formal mental health training. The intervention comprised a prerecorded audio course and an illustration-based book covering the key points from the audio sessions.

Many more RCTs on psychological interventions for psychological and psychiatric conditions have been completed in high-income countries. Published meta-analyses of RCTs have demonstrated that ACT produces clinical benefits for psychiatric conditions that are comparable to the benefits of other empirically supported cognitive-behavioral therapies (A-Tjak et al. 2015; Hayes et al. 2011). To consider one common kind of psychological outcome in crisis, patients with major depressive disorder show significant reductions in symptoms as well as improvements in quality of life following treatment with ACT (A-Tjak et al. 2018). Systematic reviews of RCTs of mindfulness-based therapies with depressive patients that focused on the specific mechanisms responsible for a change in outcome (Kazdin 2007) have shown that mindfulness (Alsubaie et al. 2017), compassion, and psychological flexibility (Gu et al. 2015) are linked to positive effects (Creswell 2017; Wielgosz et al. 2019). Reviews of RCTs on ACT interventions for individuals receiving standard treatment for psychotic disorders indicate positive effects on depression and on the frequency of hallucinations (Yıldız 2020).

No adequate measurement tool is yet available to specifically assess the process of living according to one's values (Barney et al. 2019). If, however, we take the view that living well is something more than just living without symptoms (World Health Organization 2005), it seems intuitively obvious that living according to one's values will be a key factor. More high-quality studies are needed on all types of psychological interventions and on all hypothesized mechanisms for preventing or dealing with mental suffering, and a search of the Cochrane database reveals that many such studies are on the way. Meanwhile, we may build on what is known from the many different but adjacent branches of research—on crisis, major disasters, trauma, vulnerability, resilience, posttraumatic growth, and psychological interventions for mental illnesses. Our aim in this book is to build on the available scientific evidence, the collected experience from crisis intervention, and our personal clinical experience to present a coherent new model accessible for use in the heat of the moment.

Resilience—Flexible Relating and Responding to Stress

What changes have been observed in people as they struggle with difficulties? New capacities and competences manifest in them that promote beneficial interaction with the social and physical environment and altered perspectives on life (Kalisch et al. 2017). In this way of understanding resilience, emphasis is placed on attitudes and abilities that are called upon in times of stress and distress. Some scientists have emphasized, among other things,

- Acceptance and the ability to reframe crisis as something positive, such as an opportunity for growth (Bonanno and Diminich 2013; Feder et al. 2016; Folkman and Moskowitz 2000; Tedeschi and Calhoun 2004)
- Shifting between attention to emotions in the present moment and engaging in forward-focused behavior (Bonanno 2021b; Bonanno and Diminich 2013; Folkman and Moskowitz 2004; Stroebe and Schut 1999)
- Discovering a greater meaning and purpose in life (Alim et al. 2008; Asch et al. 2021b; Feder et al. 2016; Isaacs et al. 2017; Southwick and Charney 2012b; Tsai et al. 2015)
- Connecting to one's ethics and altruistic motivations (Isaacs et al. 2017; Southwick and Charney 2012b)
- Expressing positive emotions such as gratitude, interest, love, and humor (Feder et al. 2016; Fredrickson et al. 2003; Horn et al. 2016; McGuire et al. 2021)

- Adopting positive role models (Southwick and Charney 2012b)
- Utilizing perceived social support (Alim et al. 2008; Fogle et al. 2020; Pietrzak et al. 2009; 2014; Wu et al. 2013), including emotional and practical support (Bonanno and Diminich 2013; Feder et al. 2016) and communication skills (Kalisch et al. 2017)
- Experiencing a sense of self-efficacy—trusting in your own ability to influence your destiny (Southwick et al. 2011)
- Engaging in active problem-solving (Folkman and Lazarus 1988; Southwick et al. 2005)
- Improving physical health by means of diet, exercise, and sleep (Southwick and Charney 2012a)
- Identifying cues linked to previous trauma that trigger avoidance, and introducing more positive ways of responding (Carrión and Hull 2010)
- That avoidance (e.g., denial, self-distraction, self-blame, venting), behavioral disengagement, and substances are inversely associated with positive adjustment (Alim et al. 2008; Feder et al. 2016).

To summarize, the resilience science field has moved on from the assumption that resilience is a stable personality trait—something you are, an inertia in proximity to stressors—to understanding resilience as a dynamic process of relating and responding to adversity, both during and after a crisis (Bonanno 2021b). Thus, it is better characterized as flexibility than as stability—as a willingness and ability to be internally changed by the external change that has happened. This may involve retrieving and improving a multitude of attitudes, skills, and capacities that add up to an active and resilient process in the interface between the individual and stress.

ACT Is a Translational Approach to Fostering Resilience

There is a much-discussed gap between scientific findings and the clinical interventions actually used by medical practitioners. Part of the problem is that scientific data do not always easily translate into specific guidance for the psychiatrist. Psychiatrists may be familiar with findings from resilience research but may not know how to design a clinical intervention based on those findings. The ACT approach we describe in this book is designed to bridge this gap between science and practice.

Let us start with the "stress and vulnerability model" depicted in Figure 1–2 in order to introduce a complementary understanding of the meaning of vulnerability and resilience. From an ACT perspective, the more we center on acceptance, engagement, and mindfulness, the more we increase resilience and diminish the negative impact of stress—moving toward the left in the graph. However, the more we try to eliminate distressing emotions when they arise and to choose actions by following rules, the more vulnerable we become to ending up in a crisis—moving toward the right in the graph.

From Crisis Instigation to Crisis Integration

A crisis starts with a life challenge that requires a flexible response. It does not matter who the person is or what underlying vulnerability there may be. Nor does it matter how big or small the challenge is, whether the challenge is sudden and acute or chronic and recurring, or whether the challenging event happened recently or long ago. Some challenges may require a bigger, more flexible life adaptation than other ones, but even so, the thing that determines whether a life challenge descends into a life crisis is the extent to which the person can produce a new and workable response.

As illustrated in Figure 1–3, an inflexible response is largely driven by two processes: avoidance and disengagement. *Avoidance* is trying to change and control things that cannot be changed—such as emotional and somatic responses, memories of the past, and unpleasant visions of the future. Efforts to avoid these distressing and unwanted experiences may only amplify their invasiveness and intensity, sending us into a downward spiral of feeling powerless and out of control. Attempts to avoid such experiences, paradoxically, keep us stuck in a self-perpetuating loop in which the reaction to an outer event is followed by a reaction to the reaction, and so on. *Disengagement* comes in many forms: doing more of what used to work but no longer does, keeping busy with unprioritized projects, or even withdrawal and isolation. All involve an unwillingness to approach important areas of living with the intent of solving problems and changing what can be changed. In sum, a typical crisis involves trying over and over to change what cannot be changed (negative thoughts, painful feelings, intrusive memories, bodily sensations, distressing perceptions, unwanted urges) and losing sight of what can be changed (staying present to one's experience, holding emotional pain with kindness and acceptance, connecting with personal values, one's own behavior).

This interference with the process of healing, regardless of the magnitude of the challenge, will have reached the boiling point in a typical crisis. Will we eventually change tactics, or will we continue to use a familiar, well-practiced coping strategy that is destined to fail?

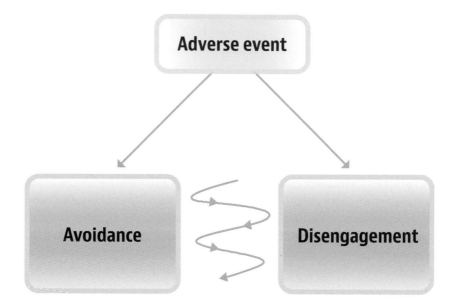

Figure 1–3.   The ACT model of crisis instigation.

If we become curious to try a flexible new response, we can do so by allowing and holding our inner responses to the present moment and choosing behavior that serves our values (Figure 1–4). This practice is both easy as pie and a locus of profound learning throughout one's lifetime. It is indeed a gradual path because we all have our own preferred avoidance strategies to which we have become accustomed. We are commonly not even aware that we are doing exactly what enables us to avoid experiencing parts, or even the whole, of our inner life. Just as prevalent is a lack of clarity about our own heartfelt values and a corresponding overreliance on rules and previously learned reactions.

A crisis signals the necessity to step out of these approaches to our inner and outer life. We have to convert avoidance into acceptance, permission, and tenderness with respect to our inner life; we have to discover our needs and deeply held values and to behave in new ways that engage with these. Integral to both acceptance and engagement is mindful present awareness; only in the present moment will we discover what is happening within and what we truly need and value. By paying attention, we can wake up to the clear distinction between elements of the crisis situation that can only be accepted and those that can be changed. We can evaluate whether our chosen actions accord with our values. Mindfulness, furthermore, provides us with the rest we need in order to strengthen our capac-

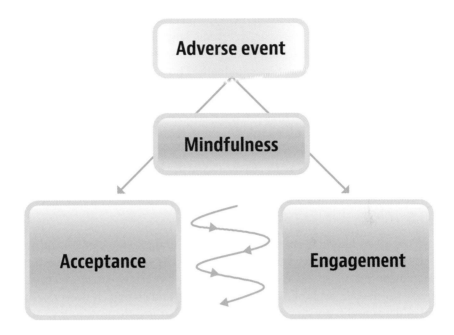

Figure 1–4. **The ACT model of crisis integration.**

ity to both hold and titrate the heartache we feel in a crisis. Sometimes just one mindful breath can provide a moment of entry into an equanimous and restful witnessing stance.

In the typical example of mourning the loss of a loved one, a flexible response means alternating between being present with the feelings of loss, emptiness, and longing and engaging in the practicalities of life without the loved one. In alternating periods of time—whether of minutes, hours, days, or weeks—we focus on tender acceptance and then on engagement with a forward focus (observe the slalom arrow in Figure 1–4). A flexible response means that we are not stuck in a rigid, repetitive pattern of avoidance and are not wed to following any particular strategy and that we can choose responses that fit the changing context. As the context shifts, so do our responses and strategies.

Often, the change required doesn't involve major leaps or radical life moves but, rather, just the opposite. Overreacting is maladaptive, and trying to immediately and completely fix everything that is broken is a recipe for failure. In crisis, very small changes of strategy practiced consistently can carry the day, even if we yearn for the magic bullet that will fix everything at once. Here, what must be learned is how to harness the strength of tiny steps when we are tempted to act in a big, impulsive way that will likely backfire. Crucial but small incremental changes—ones that alter the direction of travel—can have unexpectedly large results. Intrinsic to crisis is that the solutions to the presenting problems will not surface all at once; they will tend, rather, to emerge gradually. Thus, we may rely on patience and trust that we will know what to do when we are ready for it. Meanwhile, we relate and respond to the best of our ability. One has to "love the questions themselves," as Rainer Maria Rilke puts it in *Letters to a Young Poet*:

> Be patient toward all that is unresolved in your heart and try to love the questions themselves, like locked rooms and like books that are now written in a very foreign tongue. Do not seek the answers that cannot be given you because you would not be able to live them. And the point is, to live everything.

A crisis wisely handled can then in hindsight be appreciated as a beautiful turning point, or, better yet, a succession of several small life-changing turning points. Crisis always brings into focus important existential questions, the deeper levels of our humanity. Crisis and change, however painful and unsought, are among the main ways that people grow in love and wisdom.

The ACT Approach to Crisis— Simple but With Layers of Implication

In this book, we aim to equip the psychiatrist with a few core tools to keep in mind when supporting patients in crisis. Using the ACT crisis model, we can discern the underlying pattern of a complex crisis. When we don't know how to proceed, we will learn what is useful to focus on so that growth can be nurtured. When we have trouble reaching a patient in despair, we will practice compassion—our "capacity to remain openhearted and withstand discomfort and disquiet in the presence of pain"—and build a connection that will enable the patient and us to find the next step together (Roberts 2021). When we feel stressed about how to help a patient in dire circumstances, we will remember that the locus of control is within the patient. Instead of feeling helpless, we will be clearer that our role is to help patients bear the burdens they face. We will humbly remember that all of us have to be nudged to uncover important and timeless truths. We will patiently accept that not everything possibly helpful to the patient can be done in one fell swoop. The answers patients seek are found in harmony with life as it unfolds.

The skills to deal with crisis involve a journey of learning that never comes to an end, like learning how to find happiness or to access peace.

People can assume that such things are binary conditions—"either you're at peace or you're not"—but in reality they require practice, such that gradually one can gain ever more access to such desired states of being. From whichever point one starts, it is embedded in human beings to desire ever more ease of being, and meaning, and appreciation of life. The extent to which we stay connected to these and other values will affect the possibility of bringing them to fruition.

The appeal of the ACT model is that the skills in question are accessible and are able to facilitate lifelong, far-reaching learning for both psychiatrist and patient. Everybody experiences crises, both big ones and small ones. Our hope is that readers will be inspired to apply the ACT formula to their own lives and to model its features for their patients. Acceptance, for example, is more easily understood when the psychiatrist receives a patient who is riding the waves of desperation with tranquility and a compassionate presence than when the psychiatrist merely talks about acceptance. Our claim in this book is that crisis is an impetus to attend to one's less-than-optimal response patterns and to acquire new and flexible responses to a changed reality.

References

Acarturk C, Uygun E, Ilkkursun Z, et al: Effectiveness of a WHO self-help psychological intervention for preventing mental disorders among Syrian refugees in Turkey: a randomized controlled trial. World Psychiatry 21(1):88–95, 2022 35015365

Alim TN, Feder A, Graves RE, et al: Trauma, resilience, and recovery in a high-risk African-American population. Am J Psychiatry 165(12):1566–1575, 2008 19015233

Alsubaie M, Abbott R, Dunn B, et al: Mechanisms of action in mindfulness-based cognitive therapy (MBCT) and mindfulness-based stress reduction (MBSR) in people with physical and/or psychological conditions: a systematic review. Clin Psychol Rev 55:74–91, 2017 28501707

American Psychiatric Association: Prolonged grief disorder, in Diagnostic and Statistical Manual of Mental Disorders, 5th Edition, Text Revision. Washington, DC, American Psychiatric Publishing, 2022, pp 322–327

Asch RH, Esterlis I, Southwick SM, et al: Risk and resilience factors associated with traumatic loss-related PTSD in U.S. military veterans: results from the National Health and Resilience in Veterans Study. Psychiatry Res 298:113775, 2021a 33578060

Asch RH, Kachadourian L, Southwick SM, et al: Psychological resilience to the challenges of physical aging in older U.S. veterans: results from the 2019–2020 National Health and Resilience in Veterans Study. Am J Geriatr Psychiatry 29(12):1280–1285, 2021b 34053836

A-Tjak JG, Davis ML, Morina N, et al: A meta-analysis of the efficacy of acceptance and commitment therapy for clinically relevant mental and physical health problems. Psychother Psychosom 84(1):30–36, 2015 25547522

A-Tjak JGL, Morina N, Topper M, et al: A randomized controlled trial in routine clinical practice comparing acceptance and commitment therapy with cognitive behavioral therapy for the treatment of major depressive disorder. Psychother Psychosom 87(3):154–163, 2018 29566394

Barney JL, Lillis J, Haynos AF, et al: Assessing the valuing process in acceptance and commitment therapy: experts' review of the current status and recommendations for future measure development. J Contextual Behav Sci 12:225–233, 2019 31828006

Bonanno GA: The End of Trauma: How the New Science of Resilience Is Changing How We Think About PTSD. London, Basic Books, 2021a

Bonanno GA: The resilience paradox. Eur J Psychotraumatol 12(1):1942642, 2021b 34262670

Bonanno GA, Diminich ED: Annual Research Review: positive adjustment to adversity—trajectories of minimal-impact resilience and emergent resilience. J Child Psychol Psychiatry 54(4):378–401, 2013 23215790

Bonanno GA, Westphal M, Mancini AD: Resilience to loss and potential trauma. Annu Rev Clin Psychol 7:511–535, 2011 21091190

Bowlby J: Attachment and Loss. Vol 3: Loss, Sadness, and Depression. New York, Basic Books, 1980

Brenner AM, Coverdale J, Guerrero AP, et al: An update on trainee wellness: some progress and a long way to go. Acad Psychiatry 43:357-360, 2019

Breslau N: The epidemiology of trauma, PTSD, and other posttrauma disorders. Trauma Violence Abuse 10(3):198–210, 2009 19406860

Brumariu LE, Kerns KA: Parent-child attachment and internalizing symptoms in childhood and adolescence: a review of empirical findings and future directions. Dev Psychopathol 22(1):177–203, 2010 20102655

Bryant RA, Friedman MJ, Spiegel D, et al: A review of acute stress disorder in DSM-5. Depress Anxiety 28(9):802–817, 2011 21910186

Carkhuff BG, Berenson BG: Beyond Counseling and Therapy, 2nd Edition. New York, Holt, Rinehart, & Winston, 1977, p 165

Carrión VG, Hull K: Treatment manual for trauma-exposed youth: case studies. Clin Child Psychol Psychiatry 15(1):27–38, 2010 19914939

Carrión VG: Foreword, in Assessing and Treating Youth Exposed to Traumatic Stress. Edited by Carrión VG. Washington, DC, American Psychiatric Association Publishing, 2018, p xvii

Coverdale J, West CP, Roberts LW: Courage and mental health: physicians and physicians-in-training sharing their personal narratives. Acad Med 96(5):611–613, 2021 33885403

Creswell JD: Mindfulness interventions. Annu Rev Psychol 68:491–516, 2017 27687118

Feder A, Mota N, Salim R, et al: Risk, coping and PTSD symptom trajectories in World Trade Center responders. J Psychiatr Res 82:68–79, 2016 27468166

Fogle BM, Tsai J, Mota N, et al: The National Health and Resilience in Veterans Study: a narrative review and future directions. Front Psychiatry 11:538218, 2020 33362593

Folkman S, Lazarus RS: The relationship between coping and emotion: implications for theory and research. Soc Sci Med 26(3):309–317, 1988 3279520

Folkman S, Moskowitz JT: Positive affect and the other side of coping. Am Psychol 55(6):647–654, 2000 10892207

Folkman S, Moskowitz JT: Coping: pitfalls and promise. Annu Rev Psychol 55:745–774, 2004 14744233

Fox JH, Burkle FM Jr, Bass J, et al: The effectiveness of psychological first aid as a disaster intervention tool: research analysis of peer-reviewed literature from 1990-2010. Disaster Med Public Health Prep 6(3):247–252, 2012 23077267

Fredrickson BL, Tugade MM, Waugh CE, et al: What good are positive emotions in crises? A prospective study of resilience and emotions following the terrorist attacks on the United States on September 11th, 2001. J Pers Soc Psychol 84(2):365–376, 2003 12585810

Gradus JL, Qin P, Lincoln AK, et al: The association between adjustment disorder diagnosed at psychiatric treatment facilities and completed suicide. Clin Epidemiol 2:23–28, 2010 20865099

Greenberg N, Docherty M, Gnanapragasam S, et al: Managing mental health challenges faced by healthcare workers during covid-19 pandemic. BMJ 368:m1211, 2020 32217624

Griffin BJ, Purcell N, Burkman K, et al: Moral injury: an integrative review. J Trauma Stress 32(3):350–362, 2019 30688367

Gu J, Strauss C, Bond R, et al: How do mindfulness-based cognitive therapy and mindfulness-based stress reduction improve mental health and wellbeing? A systematic review and meta-analysis of mediation studies. Clin Psychol Rev 37:1–12, 2015 25689576

Guterres A: Opening remarks at virtual press encounter to launch the report on the Socio-Economic Impacts of COVID-19. March 31, 2020. Available at: https://www.un.org/sg/en/content/sg/speeches/2020-03-31/remarks-launch-of-report-the-socio-economic-impacts-of-covid-19. Accessed August 22, 2020.

Haglund A, Lysell H, Larsson H, et al: Suicide immediately after discharge from psychiatric inpatient care: a cohort study of nearly 2.9 million discharges. J Clin Psychiatry 80(2):80, 2019 30758922

Hailes HP, Yu R, Danese A, et al: Long-term outcomes of childhood sexual abuse: an umbrella review. Lancet Psychiatry 6(10):830–839, 2019 31519507

Harper D: Crisis. Etymonline, 2020. Available at: https://www.etymonline.com/word/crisis. Accessed September 1, 2020.

Harvey AG, Bryant RA: Acute stress disorder: a synthesis and critique. Psychol Bull 128(6):886–902, 2002 12405136

Hayes SC, Strosahl KD, Wilson KG: Acceptance and Commitment Therapy: An Experiential Approach to Behavior Change. New York, Guilford, 1999

Hayes SC, Villatte M, Levin M, et al: Open, aware, and active: contextual approaches as an emerging trend in the behavioral and cognitive therapies. Annu Rev Clin Psychol 7:141–168, 2011 21219193

Hobfoll SE, Mancini AD, Hall BJ, et al: The limits of resilience: distress following chronic political violence among Palestinians. Soc Sci Med 72(8):1400–1408, 2011 21440348

Horn SR, Charney DS, Feder A: Understanding resilience: new approaches for preventing and treating PTSD. Exp Neurol 284(Pt B):119–132, 2016 27417856

Isaacs K, Mota NP, Tsai J, et al: Psychological resilience in U.S. military veterans: a 2-year, nationally representative prospective cohort study. J Psychiatr Res 84:301–309, 2017 27814502

James RK, Gilliland BE: Crisis Intervention Strategies, 7th Edition. Belmont, CA, Cengage Learning, 2012, p 8

Kalisch R, Baker DG, Basten U, et al: The resilience framework as a strategy to combat stress-related disorders. Nat Hum Behav 1(11):784–790, 2017 31024125

Kantamneni N: The impact of the COVID-19 pandemic on marginalized populations in the United States: a research agenda. J Vocat Behav 119:103439, 2020 32390658

Kazdin AE: Mediators and mechanisms of change in psychotherapy research. Annu Rev Clin Psychol 3:1–27, 2007 17716046

Klein N: The Shock Doctrine: The Rise of Disaster Capitalism. London, Penguin Books, 2008

Lee PH, Anttila V, Won H, et al: Genomic relationships, novel loci, and pleiotropic mechanisms across eight psychiatric disorders. Cell 179(7):1469–1482, 2019 31835028

McGuire AP, Fogle BM, Tsai J, et al: Dispositional gratitude and mental health in the U.S. veteran population: results from the National Health and Resilience Veterans Study. J Psychiatr Res 135:279–288, 2021 33516080

Mustak S: Climate change and disaster-induced displacement in the global south: a review, in Climate Change, Disaster and Adaptations: Contextualising Human Responses to Ecological Change. Edited by Siddiqui AR, Sahay A. Cham, Switzerland, Springer International Publishing, 2022, pp 107–120

Norris FH, Tracy M, Galea S: Looking for resilience: understanding the longitudinal trajectories of responses to stress. Soc Sci Med 68(12):2190–2198, 2009 19403217

North CS, Pfefferbaum B: Mental health response to community disasters: a systematic review. JAMA 310(5):507–518, 2013 23925621

Pietrzak RH, Johnson DC, Goldstein MB, et al: Psychosocial buffers of traumatic stress, depressive symptoms, and psychosocial difficulties in veterans of Operations Enduring Freedom and Iraqi Freedom: the role of resilience, unit support, and postdeployment social support. J Spec Oper Med 9(3):74–78, 2009 19739480

Pietrzak RH, Feder A, Singh R, et al: Trajectories of PTSD risk and resilience in World Trade Center responders: an 8-year prospective cohort study. Psychol Med 44(1):205–219, 2014 23551932

Prigerson HG, Kakarala S, Gang J, et al: History and status of prolonged grief disorder as a psychiatric diagnosis. Annu Rev Clin Psychol 17:109–126, 2021 33524263

Roberts LW: Advancing understanding of compassion and compassion training. Acad Med 96(7):929–930, 2021 34183476

Rohde N, Tang KK, Osberg L, et al: The effect of economic insecurity on mental health: recent evidence from Australian panel data. Soc Sci Med 151:250–258, 2016 26826683

Roth TL, Sweatt JD: Annual Research Review: epigenetic mechanisms and environmental shaping of the brain during sensitive periods of development. J Child Psychol Psychiatry 52(4):398–408, 2011 20626526

Southwick SM, Vythilingam M, Charney DS: The psychobiology of depression and resilience to stress: implications for prevention and treatment. Annu Rev Clin Psychol 1:255–91, 2005

Southwick SM, Litz BT, Charney D, et al: Resilience and Mental Health: Challenges Across the Lifespan. Cambridge, UK, Cambridge University Press, 2011

Southwick SM, Charney DS: The science of resilience: implications for the prevention and treatment of depression. Science 338(6103):79–82, 2012a 23042887

Southwick SM, Charney DS: Resilience: The Science of Mastering Life's Greatest Challenges. Cambridge, UK, Cambridge University Press, 2012b

Southwick SM, Bonanno GA, Masten AS, et al: Resilience definitions, theory, and challenges: interdisciplinary perspectives. Eur J Psychotraumatol 5:5, 2014 25317257

Stroebe M, Schut H: The dual process model of coping with bereavement: rationale and description. Death Stud 23(3):197–224, 1999 10848151

Strosahl KD, Robinson PJ, Gustavsson T: Brief Interventions for Radical Change: Principles and Practice of Focused Acceptance and Commitment Therapy. Oakland, CA, New Harbinger Publications, 2012

Tedeschi RG, Calhoun LG: Target Article: Posttraumatic growth: conceptual foundations and empirical evidence. Psychol Inq 15(1):1–18, 2004

Tol WA, Barbui C, Galappatti A, et al: Mental health and psychosocial support in humanitarian settings: linking practice and research. Lancet 378(9802):1581–1591, 2011 22008428

Tol WA, Leku MR, Lakin DP, et al: Guided self-help to reduce psychological distress in South Sudanese female refugees in Uganda: a cluster randomised trial. Lancet Glob Health 8(2):e254–e263, 2020 31981556

Tsai J, El-Gabalawy R, Sledge WH, et al: Post-traumatic growth among veterans in the USA: results from the National Health and Resilience in Veterans Study. Psychol Med 45(1):165–179, 2015 25065450

Turecki G, Brent DA: Suicide and suicidal behaviour. Lancet 387(10024):1227–1239, 2016 26385066

Widom CS, Czaja SJ, Kozakowski SS, et al: Does adult attachment style mediate the relationship between childhood maltreatment and mental and physical health outcomes? Child Abuse Negl 76:533–545, 2018 28522128

Wielgosz J, Goldberg SB, Kral TRA, et al: Mindfulness meditation and psychopathology. Annu Rev Clin Psychol 15:285–316, 2019 30525995

World Health Organization: Promoting Mental Health: Concepts, Emerging Evidence, Practice. Geneva, World Health Organization, 2005

Wu G, Feder A, Cohen H, et al: Understanding resilience. Front Behav Neurosci 7:10, 2013 23422934

Yeager K, Roberts A (eds): Crisis Intervention Handbook: Assessment, Treatment, and Research. New York, Oxford University Press, 2015

Yıldız E: The effects of acceptance and commitment therapy in psychosis treatment: a systematic review of randomized controlled trials. Perspect Psychiatr Care 56(1):149–167, 2020 31074039

Zisook S, Shear K: Grief and bereavement: what psychiatrists need to know. World Psychiatry 8(2):67–74, 2009 19516922

Zubin J, Spring B: Vulnerability: a new view of schizophrenia. J Abnorm Psychol 86(2):103–126, 1977 858828

The ACT Model of Crisis Instigation

Chaos may rattle you, but order can kill you.

—Ajahn Sucitto*

Crisis Instigation: A Neuroscience and Behavior-Analytic Perspective

The ubiquity of crises should not be attributed solely to the fact that life challenges, including extreme ones, are a prevalent part of human existence. This chapter describes something even more ubiquitous, something that seems so natural and innocent as to be taken for granted but, unless we become aware of it, can become a millstone around our neck in challenging times. This something is integral to the way we are shaped by evolution in interplay with our individual developmental circumstances, but it need not control our responses. It has to do with how we perceive the world—both inner and outer—and how we learn about and manage our responses to it. Through discovering our inherent tendencies, we become free to consider and adopt other, more beneficial responses to crisis that will facilitate healing and favorable outcomes in our mind, emotions, and body—and in our life as a whole.

We use the term *crisis instigation* to encompass the processes by which an individual responds to a challenge, no matter how small or large,

---

* From Lindeblad 2022.

that ratchet up their suffering to crisis levels. As this term suggests, a crisis does not come in a bottle; it is created via a dynamic, iterative process that occurs within the individual and between the individual and their surrounding life context. This dynamic, iterative interaction is rich in opportunities for the psychiatrist to interrupt the downward spiral of crisis response.

The source of trouble when we deal with challenges is the combination of avoiding our inner emotional and physical responses and acting according to insidious habits based on previous learning. The crisis formula introduced in Chapter 1, "Crisis Fundamentals," comprises, in short, a precipitating challenging and painful event and a response to this that is characterized by two processes that we call "avoidance" and "disengagement." Before we examine helpful ways of moving through hardships, we must first begin to unpack these problematic processes. In order to fully understand them, we examine the questions of how and why they arise. In the next section, we briefly survey these questions from a neuroscience and behavior-analytic perspective.

Evolution-Shaped Learning

Integrated in the central neural system of human beings are a few principal ways of perceiving events, learning about them, and guiding our behavior in response. The very existence of a neural system means that perception, for example, is not a simple reflection of the environment; it is a synthesis of presently incoming information and of prior knowledge already integrated in the system that processes this new input (Carlsson et al. 2000; Frith 2007; Frith and Dolan 1997). Prior knowledge certainly derives from the individual's previous experience, but what may not always be realized is that *how* we perceive, as well as *how* we learn and behave, has evolved from a long sequence of forerunners whose brains were shaped by evolutionary processes. This learning by our ancestors has already taken place. Our brains have been shaped through phylogenesis and incorporate innate knowledge.

Through evolution, we have acquired competence to respond to significant stimuli on an approach–avoidance continuum. We have inherited *approach* responses to "primary rewards," also called "primary reinforcers" (e.g., food, water, safety, care), just as we have inherited *avoidance* responses in relation to "primary punishments" (e.g., pain, specific dangers). At a basic level, stimuli of primary positive or negative value guide our choices of approach or withdrawal, akin to a flower's turning toward the sun and away from the shade. In organisms with a central neural system, the approach or withdrawal response has an experiential aspect. Emotional experiences and responses indicate the positive or negative value of external stimuli and provide the motivational force for human behavior (Damasio 1999; Dolan 2002; LeDoux 1998).

The human neural system is thus wired to detect a snake with alacrity and to then evoke physiological responses of raised heartbeat and sweaty hands, detect this physiological body state, and produce behavior to help the individual escape the situation. This is all part of the emotional response of fear. Emotions are the result of linking such stimuli to behavior that helped our ancestors to construct circumstances advantageous to survival and to transmitting their genes down the generations (Carlsson et al. 2004; Öhman et al. 2007). That is why we are inherently more afraid of snakes than of traffic or of handling broken electrical devices; only in recent generations have the latter experiences become more prevalent and caused far more deaths.

Model-Free Learning

Higher-order organisms have, as an implemented function of their brains, the ability to learn throughout their respective lifetimes. This capacity for learning enables survival in different environments—not only that of one's ancestors—and adaptability to innumerable new situations. One way to learn in real time is from the *consequences* of our own behavior, often described as based on "trial and error." Certain actions that have certain consequences will affect how we respond to similar situations in the future.

A reward serves as a "positive reinforcer"—that is, it increases the likelihood that a behavior will occur. Positive reinforcement occurs when something desirable is presented as a consequence of a behavior, just as a "reward" is a particular object or experience you receive after you've done something well (Schultz 2006). Negative reinforcement, on the other hand, occurs when something unpleasant is removed as a consequence of a behavior. Both types of reinforcement involve consequences that *increase* the likelihood of approach and avoidance behaviors. The word *positive* implies adding, and the word *negative* implies removing. Positive reinforcement encourages behavior that *adds* something desirable; negative reinforcement encourages behavior that *removes* something undesirable. Distinct from these are *punishments*—undesirable consequences to behavior that tend to decrease that behavior and increase it when removed.

We can also *associate* events in time and space, such as when Ivan Pavlov's dog learned to salivate (i.e., a response) upon hearing the sound of a bell, after several trials of first hearing a bell and then being given a bowl of food. The bell became in this way also a "secondary reinforcer": the neutral sound of the bell was linked to the primary positive reinforcer, the food. Both humans and animals rely on learning from consequences and from associations, and this allows them to engage in fairly complex patterns of behavior. In the human brain, such learning commonly involves subcortical areas, but it is also a capacity of animals with smaller brains than ours.

Although learning about associations and consequences in these ways can be precise and adaptive and allow *some* flexibility, it suffers from two great flaws. First, it is still pretty inflexible. For example, behavior learned through trial and error is commonly built into the neural system in the form of direct connections between stimuli and responses, such that the presentation of a stimulus automatically elicits a habitual response. This type of reinforcement learning essentially forms reflexes that can be difficult to suppress when the response in question is inappropriate. Such learning does not require an internal model, explicit knowledge, or conscious experience of either the stimuli or of the response and its consequence. It has therefore been called *model-free learning*. Second, it is slow. The human or animal must learn about the rewards and punishments through direct personal experience (Frith 2021; Huys et al. 2014). Thus, model-free learning does not fully explain how we can create and operate within the complex milieus we inhabit.

Model-Based Learning

On top of the model-free learning systems, the brains of both humans and animals have access to a far more flexible learning system: learning based on internal models of the world. Whereas model-free systems involve learning about rewards through trial and error and associations, model-based systems involve learning about the world. *Model-based learning* still evaluates the value of one's actions, but it does so based on internal models of objects, events, responses, and anticipated future outcomes. Internal models can be based on our own memories of experiences or can be conveyed by others. Models can be used to choose our own responses to situations never previously encountered that have similarities to situations experienced by others. Models thus liberate organisms from being in thrall to automatic responses to immediate circumstances. In the human brain, models are processed mainly on the cortical level (Frith 2021; McClure et al. 2004). Comparisons of situations now and then and of actions that have previously led to a rewarding experience enable time-efficient learning in relation to complex matters. What's more, model-based learning can be verbally communicated (Frith 2021).

Rule-Governed Behavior and Language

Language can be used to communicate many different types of models that advance our understanding of the world and of ourselves. A model-based system creates an inner representation of aspects of the world, such as a tree, and language connects the word *tree* to this inner representation. Words are, in turn, linked to other words, creating bigger, more complex models of the world. By combining and connecting bits of information—mentally comparing things, identifying similarities and distinctions, recognizing correlations and conditionalities, categorizing, taking alternative perspectives, predicting consequences—we obtain models about the world that further down the line have enabled us, for example, to navigate across oceans. The power of language is that it is largely based upon arbitrarily derived stimulus relations (Hayes et al. 2001). To "derive relations arbitrarily" means that anything can be related to anything else. *Relating*, in turn, simply means responding to one thing in terms of another, such as when we evaluate something as "more rewarding" by relating it to something "less rewarding."

Freed from having to learn about the world through trial and error, humans can play with models, both verbal and nonverbal, of the world around them using imagination, guesswork, evaluation, recall, and a thousand other modes of cognition. The ensuing combinations of stimulus relations then directly regulate the specified behavior through "rules." Verbal rules can thus be understood within a behavior-analytic framework of learning about associations and consequences without having to learn through direct experience (Villatte et al. 2019).

ACT is unique in the field of evidence-based psychotherapy in that many of its core principles derive from a behavior-analytic account of human language known as *relational frame theory* (RFT) (Hayes et al. 2001). For three decades, RFT research has delved into the *functions* of human language as a system of behavioral control. This research tradition has demonstrated that language is responsible both for our most powerful forms of problem-solving and for our most powerful and enduring forms of dysfunction and suffering.

An intrinsic degree of risk exists in a system that allows us to relate anything to anything else without first having to establish the currency and validity of that linkage through direct experience. Language and all other forms of symbolic activity that elaborate upon models, whether spoken or experienced as thoughts, images, sounds, somatic sensations, and emotions, are a source not only of human resilience but also of human frailty.

In this book, we are particularly interested in one specific function of language: that of promoting social organization. It has even been suggested that the evolutionary advantage of learning with the help of language is directly tied to the fact that this is a powerful way to create complex social systems and cultural practices (Nowak et al. 2010). Social and cultural knowledge are also conveyed through model-free learning, as well as learning based on nonverbal models and symbols. Language, however, strengthens the process and allows us to both organize and execute specific behavioral sequences according to increasingly complex social requirements. Development from infancy to adulthood involves acquiring these complex kinds of rules for behavior. As we grow up, we come to depend less on external monitoring and guidance in order both to flourish and to comply with social norms; we are progressively more governed by an internalized, rule-following process known as "self-instructional control" (Goubert et al. 2020). People essentially use language as a means to implement self-instructions that are programmed through their social training.

Benefits of Rule-Governed Behavior

Complex, organized sequences of behaviors under self-instructional control are an important part of rule-governed behavior. Rule-governed behavior based on language typically contains many individual behavioral units; the execution of these individual units leads in aggregate to a socially sanctioned result. Rule-governed behavior allows lengthy behavioral sequences to be performed without any immediate external reward (Goubert et al. 2020). Through imagination, the future reward (or punishment) is experienced in the present and thus serves to foster desired socially defined outcomes long into the future. With the help of inner models, distant consequences of rewards and punishments are brought into the present to help us direct our behavior toward advantageous consequences that we would not otherwise attain. The most distinctive features of problem-solving, goal-directed behavior, and complex social systems are intimately tied to this type of rule governance (including studying for years to get a degree in medicine or other health services profession!).

Risks of Relying on Previous Learning

The methods of learning just discussed help us to function. Sometimes, however, when we behave in compliance with previous learning, whether shaped by evolution or by model-free or model-based learning, we find ourselves in trouble. The key word here is "previous." A significantly changed situation often requires a new response. If nothing else, a crisis is certainly a new situation that requires a new set of responses from the individual.

Let's consider an example of evolution-shaped learning For 10,000 generations, fat and sugar were exceptionally valuable in promoting survival and thus became a potent primary reinforcer of approach behavior. However, for the past few generations, fat and sugar have been available at every turn in some parts of the world, and excessive consumption of them is becoming a major cause of sickness and death. Complications will similarly arise when people rely automatically on other instances of previous learning.

Luckily, humans have at their disposal some higher-order capacities for perception and learning—that is, metacognitive and meta-awareness abilities. In Part II we explore in detail the powerful implications of these most recently evolved learning systems. The prefix *meta-* comes from the Greek for "beyond" or "with" and is used to indicate a concept that transcends another particular concept. With these higher-order abilities, seemingly unique to the human species (Frith 2021), we can become aware of the urges, models, and rules that may have served well in previous situations but no longer do so. In *metacognition*—cognition about cognition—an individual can reflect on the rules or models that guide their behavior. With *meta-awareness*, they can observe and receive emotions, rules, and thoughts as just that, which with time will make them less compelling. These meta-abilities also allow exploration of deeper long-term values to guide behavior. They provide the foundation for mindfulness, acceptance, and engagement and are crucial to flexibility during crisis. Before we get into that, let us first unpack how crisis is instigated by reliance on previous learning.

Crisis Instigation Through Disengagement

From a behaviorist perspective, the significance of any given behavior can be gauged only with respect to its context. A behavior that was effective in some previous context may have disastrous consequences when exercised in a slightly different context. Internal rules shaped in previous contexts may be misaligned with new circumstances; obedience to these rules may therefore lead to *disengagement* from the circumstances. We argue that this is one of two principal ways—the other being *avoidance*—in which people can slip into crisis following a catastrophe or major change in their life. Avoidance and disengagement often go hand in hand in the process of crisis instigation. Here, for the sake of clarity, we describe them separately to distinguish what exactly is going on that is unhelpful.

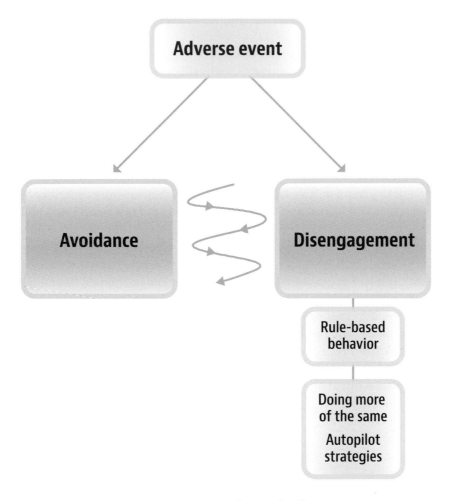

Figure 2–1.   Crisis instigation through disengagement.

   We use *disengagement* as an umbrella term for choosing actions based on previous learning instead of engaging with what this new turn in life actually asks us to do. The common denominator of disengaged behavior is compliance with previously learned and self-instructional rules and the lack of ability, knowledge, or motivation to engage with present circumstances and the real consequences of one's behavior. In crisis, disengagement typically manifests as repetitive use of a limited behavioral repertoire—taking the same action despite evidence that this action is patently ineffective or even counterproductive (Figure 2–1).

   As we've seen, language-based rules serve to promote a social group that is organized and behaves in largely predictable ways. Language pro-

vides a huge evolutionary advantage in protecting the group from preda-
tors, promoting procreation, and sustaining order (Nowak et al. 2010).
The kinds of rules an individual learns during their developmental years
to ensure safety through belonging to the group are those most deeply in-
grained and most difficult to question. (Rules learned about algebra are
more easily forgotten!) We live much of our lives inside this personally
tailored system of rules, whose ever-present regulatory functions are almost invisible to us. However, we may be aware at some level that much
of our behavior is ultimately linked to a wish for approval, inclusion, respect, and even love within our social group, as well as being oriented toward safety and survival. The rules we learned growing up are often along
the lines of "In order to be loved, included, or safe, I have to achieve or be
perfect; be special, needed, strong, or self-reliant; or acquire knowledge
so I can predict events, fit in and not stand out, or avoid expressing anger."

Everyone has their own intricate set of rules that worked within the
immediate family environment in which they grew up. Behavior based on
this rule matrix is in many ways functional and has gotten us far, but at
some point, and specifically in a crisis, we will be forced to investigate the
validity and currency of these rules.

Context Insensitivity and Adaptive Peaks

One dangerous feature of behavior that is guided by self-instructional
rules is that it diminishes the individual's sensitivity to actual real-world
outcomes. Imagined rewards or punishments prevail over actual consequences. This tendency, also known as *context insensitivity* (Goubert et al.
2020), indicates that rule-governed behavior is very resistant to change,
even when the consequences of following the rules are negative. For example, people in crisis often find it difficult to stop or to change ineffective
coping strategies if those strategies are governed by rules. As an example,
if a previous consequence, "C-old" (receiving approval and safety), has
been the result of behavior "B" (working long hours, never giving up), but
what actually occurs is a new, unwanted consequence, "C-new" (symptoms of burnout and ill-health), there is no guarantee that the derived relationship B→C-old (hard work→approval and survival) will be modified
to consider C-new.

There are several mechanisms through which arbitrarily derived rules
prevent us from learning directly from real consequences. First, a rule entails not only the promised positive consequences for following it but also
the aversive consequences of not following it. Moreover, the *imagined*
consequences of breaking a rule are generally seen as worse than the *actual* consequences, because the influence of rules can be "augmented," or

strengthened, through association with additional desirable or undesirable social consequences. In the earlier C-old/C-new example, a new response of taking breaks and generally allowing more time for rest will evoke feelings not only of resistance but likely also of discomfort. This discomfort is connected to the rule's intrinsic specification of what will happen if it's not followed. The model that safety and love are found through achievement and work implies that unsafety and rejection will follow from "slacking" (a possible rule-based word for resting and recovering). Although this rule may have been true in the past, it should be questioned to better serve one's freedom of choice, one's health, and possibly even one's survival. New learning involves riding waves of fear about the imagined rejection that is part of one's rule system—and about dealing with reactions and reprimands from colleagues and institutions guided by similar rules—before that rule will loosen its grip.

Another feature of rule-governed behavior that leads to context insensitivity is the sheer volume of rules that humans must follow to participate in the social order. Given the brain's limited information-processing capacity, it is far more efficient to remove voluntary control from the equation and to engage in behavioral sequences, even complex ones, more or less automatically. A vast proportion of everyday sequences of behavior is under the control of environmental cues (Kahneman 2011; Vatansever et al. 2017). Thus, automatic rule-following is our default mode of operating in the world. However, it does not need to be. Many of the mindfulness and perspective-taking techniques used in ACT are designed to bring patients off autopilot mode so they can see their nonverbal and verbally constructed rules from an observer perspective instead of a participant perspective. They are then freed from having to follow rules that don't work.

One more characteristic of context-insensitive, rule-governed behavior is that it brings about "adaptive peaks." These are advantageous results of a behavior that fails to provide a platform for future development (Villatte et al. 2019). Working long hours and never giving up may have gotten us far and may therefore seem a logical behavior to pursue. In reality, that rule has brought an adaptive peak that is conducive neither to the improvement of behavioral choices nor to insights about safety and love, or it may have brought about limited success relating only to one area in life (e.g., one's working life but not one's love life) and will, in time, need to be investigated from a new angle.

Escalating symptoms of burnout make it clear that behavior based on old models, previous learning, previous consequences, and outdated rules will not provide the solution to all situations. Sometimes we find ourselves doing more of the same things that brought us into the troubled situation in the first place: when fatigued, we may work slower and our decision processes may become more arduous. To compensate, we may put in even more hours and thereby squeeze out the very thing—rest—that could ameliorate the problem and establish a new equilibrium. As Chapter 7, "Engagement," will elucidate, the new response that will provide us a way out is commonly the one response we resist the most. What is needed is a flexible, experimental approach that allows new responses to be formed in light of present consequences and of personal values, such as better health. This behavior will be engendered with awareness of inner values and with close attention to external consequences. Such "mindful doing" contrasts with "unmindful doing"—a disengaged, autopilot strategy of business as usual.

One last peril of rule governance concerns the ability to relate anything to anything else. Language not only allows us to learn from one another and from memories of previous experiences but also enables the creation of networks of relations that we have never been taught or experienced. We can in this way arbitrarily alter how objects, situations, and events impact our thoughts, feelings, and actions. We can amplify our level of subjective distress through relating one distressing subjective experience to another one in the past—or to one that has yet to happen. In other words, after a painful life experience that precipitates a natural psychological response, our reactions can be linked to other events in numerous ways, even in ways unrelated to the original situation. Within our minds, we may verbally associate previously learned distress related to one stimulus with other, more innocuous stimuli and thereby extend pain to ever larger areas of our life. This feature of language is so powerful that even positive life experiences can be related to negative ones and thereby be converted into difficult experiences. We can be transported anywhere at the speed of thought without moving a muscle. This capacity opens up a huge range of possibilities, but it also provides a broad and ubiquitous interface with pain and suffering and an easy pathway into crisis.

In sum, although rule-governed behavior is a fantastic evolutionary accomplishment and does much to increase our effectiveness in choosing and guiding behavior, it has limitations. In times of significant change or crisis, following rules will not work and can actually make things worse. In dealing with crisis situations, it is therefore crucial for the individual to learn to spot disengagement and to let go of rules that no longer work.

Psychiatric practice resembles detective work in that it makes a big difference if you know what you're looking for. The dialogues that follow illustrate the process of probing for unworkable underlying rules, and for other factors contributing to a crisis's development, without any intention to intervene—yet. In the first two cases, we describe certain rule-governed processes that contributed to the crisis in question. The first case concerns a crisis at a fairly early stage; the second is one in which rule governance has aggravated the situation over some years.

David: Clinical Dialogue on Crisis Instigation With Disengagement at an Early Stage

David, a 35-year-old married man with two children 10 and 12 years old, had been physically very active in his free time, practicing several sports and coaching his children's basketball teams. Seven weeks ago, he was badly injured in a bicycle race and sustained a spinal cord injury that left him able to use his arms but not his legs. Since the accident, he has only desultorily engaged with his rehabilitation program and has been irritable and short with his wife and medical staff. The lives of husband and wife have been very different these past 7 weeks; David's wife has to do the parenting and take care of the household on top of her full-time job, and she is also dealing with the problem of how to rearrange the house to accommodate a wheelchair.

Meanwhile, David, residing at the inpatient rehabilitation facility, has a lot of time on his own as he faces his painful and disturbing new situation. He has let one of the nurses know that he is considering a divorce. The staff have been struggling to motivate him to engage in the rehabilitation program and have been unable to make him understand the need to wait before contemplating such big decisions as divorce. The clinical team has referred him to an in-house psychiatrist.

In this first meeting with David, and later in two other cases, we begin to get a sense of how the tool of acceptance can be applied in crisis consultations. Rules are designed to gain something that's valued as well as to avoid something bad, and acceptance processes will therefore be beneficial when they connect to such valued things and will often reveal the rules pertaining to them. Acceptance is explored in more depth in later chapters; the focus in the dialogue here is primarily on figuring out the prevailing rules guiding David in relating to his new situation.

Psychiatrist: I've been asked to come and see you. I'm a psychiatrist consultant. The staff here seem to be worried about you.
David: Well, *I* certainly haven't asked you to come.
Psychiatrist: Would you still allow for me to stay for a while?
David: (*silence*) Nobody needs to worry about me.
Psychiatrist: I see…. May I still stay?
David: (*silence*)
Psychiatrist: I understand that you had a very bad accident 7 weeks ago?
David: No need to remind me.
Psychiatrist: It makes perfect sense to me that you should be angry. Who wouldn't?

To seek connection, the psychiatrist begins where the patient is, reflecting the feeling tone of his first remarks. When their feeling of anger is reflected to them, some will feel heard, whereas others, having a rule that one shouldn't be angry, will object but may provide another feeling word (e.g., "hopeless" or "scared") that the psychiatrist can then reflect back. David responds again with silence.

> Psychiatrist: I don't think anybody could imagine what it would be like to face the fact of never being able to walk again, until they've experienced it firsthand.

The psychiatrist is reflecting the possible feeling of experiential loneliness implied in David's "Nobody needs to worry about me."

> David: That's quite right—nobody understands. And nobody will ever understand. That includes you, by the way.
> Psychiatrist: Would you nevertheless let me share your company for a while?
> David: I'm tired. I've just come back from lunch, which is a hassle just to get there and back. I can't even carry my own tray! How long are you going to stay?
> Psychiatrist: (*silence*) I'll take that as a yes. Psychiatrists are rarely fully welcomed.

The psychiatrist does not respond directly to David's question, guessing that he is trying to push away company as an avoidance strategy.

> Psychiatrist: I'm guessing from what you say that it would be nice if somebody could understand, or at least hear, some of what you're up against?

The psychiatrist chooses to stay with the topic of understanding because David responded to it. Although David spoke of a lack of understanding, the psychiatrist phrases the need for understanding in positive terms to help David connect to this value.

> David: Yeah, right?! But who could? And it wouldn't actually help anyway.
> Psychiatrist: Things seem pointless…

She reflects what he has expressed, staying with what comes up, modeling acceptance of what is here at each step of the process.

> David: Totally…. I see no point in anything.

They are on a roll: connection is beginning to happen. In moving on, the psychiatrist keeps in mind that the task is not to get the patient to feel differently, to fix or to change him, but to be present with him when he is thinking what he is thinking and feeling what he is feeling and to provide awareness and acceptance of all of that.

> Psychiatrist: I heard you're even considering a divorce.
> David: (*silence*) We're becoming more distant from one another. She shows no sign of understanding or of listening to what I'm going through.
> Psychiatrist: And that's what you actually need most at the moment—someone to stay and listen to the enormity of it all.
> David: She really doesn't need a cripple to take care of on top of everything. I don't want to be a burden to her. I won't accept that.
> Psychiatrist: I hear two quite painful words here: "cripple" and "burden."

Instead of arguing with and correcting David, the psychiatrist repeats these words to lift them into his present-moment awareness. Because he is moving close to his self-instructional rules, there's a good chance he's not even aware that they're influencing his behavior.

> David: (*silence*) Yeah. Quite.
> Psychiatrist: I can imagine many feelings and needs related to those words. You truly want to contribute on an equal basis in your marriage but just don't know what that would look like. Is that right?

She focuses on David's values (to contribute) rather than on his thoughts ("she doesn't need a cripple") because the levels of emotion and values are where acceptance is most crucial at this point.

> David: She needs a man, not someone in a wheelchair who needs attention and help doing just about anything. I have nothing to offer to her—other than problems.
> Psychiatrist: Nothing to offer.... Another painful thought. What stands behind it? Fear of not being enough? Fear of not being loved if you can't now offer what you used to?

Again, the psychiatrist is inviting awareness around the thought and exploring underlying feelings and needs. Some of David's rules around love are surfacing.

> David: How could I possibly be.... How could we possibly love each other from here on?
> Psychiatrist: (*Silence*) Ah, the pain of imagining the loss of love. A painful thought, for sure, which connects to one of life's great mysteries—the question of where love resides.

Landing here, providing awareness and acceptance, welcoming this fear and the value of love into the dialogue, invites the patient to be with these for a while before the conversation continues. We return to this unfolding dialogue in Chapter 3, "The ACT Model of Crisis Integration." For now, the psychiatrist has enough information to form a hypothesis about the rules obstructing David from moving on in this crisis situation. There is nothing wrong with the values of love and of contributing, but David's rules for how to fulfill those values are blocking him from engaging with the changed situation. The rules in question are probably along the lines of "In order to be loved I have to achieve and to contribute in a practical and monetary way" and "In order to be the man in a marriage, I must be physically fit and fully functioning sexually." Unable any longer to adhere to these rules the way he used to, David is exposed to the fear of losing love, but he is dodging that fear as best he can by using the avoidance strategy of pushing his partner away first. Here is an example of how avoidance and disengagement go hand in hand: David is avoiding the experience of fear by pushing his loved ones away, and he is disengaging from the difficult new situation by holding back from both his rehabilitation and his family. He very likely has other rules as well that prevent him from making favorable decisions at this turning point in his life. It's not terribly important for the psychiatrist to precisely identify the best-fitting rule. What matters is the process of facilitating the emergence of rules into awareness and promoting connection to underlying values.

Another thing we could infer from David's situation is that the rule "In order to be loved I have to achieve and to contribute in a practical and monetary way" has reached an adaptive peak. To move on, David will have to find new ways of understanding love. Right now, he may not be able to perceive his rule very clearly, and it will make little sense to spell it out to him at this point. It would probably just make him angry again instead of giving him the chance to feel his underlying fear. When we come back to his process in Chapter 3, we also discuss the crucial distinction between values and rules.

For some, like David, life can be relatively tranquil until it is suddenly disrupted or even shattered by events beyond one's control. Others, meanwhile, live in highly unstable circumstances presenting recurrent major challenges, in which small additional changes can unsettle one's equilibrium on an almost-daily basis. In psychiatry, we see patients occupying all points along this continuum, with a bias toward those on the latter end. Although David provides a typical example of a crisis, he is not a typical patient in psychiatric care, although with time he could become one if he does not shift strategies. Let us, then, introduce a second case study from a psychiatric outpatient care unit.

Anton: Clinical Dialogue on Crisis Instigation With Disengagement at a Late Stage

Anton was a 28-year-old man, now single, who has a 7-year-old daughter. He grew up with his mother, twin sister, and stepfather, but as a child he had to take care of himself quite a lot. The stepfather wasn't good to the twins, so they both moved far away at the age of 16. Anton reconnected at that time with his biological father, who taught Anton his craft, heavy mechanical work, and thus helped him mature into a skilled and capable working man. He met a woman with whom he had a daughter, but their relationship was stormy, and they separated 2 years ago. Since then, Anton had been struggling for shared custody of their daughter, a matter not yet settled when Anton first came for psychiatry. Also hanging over him was the threat that he would lose his apartment because of unpaid bills. He had the money but had always lacked the initiative to open mail and pay bills. He was drinking quite a bit, but not excessively. Over the past 9 months he had become increasingly depressed, and lately he had been struggling with intense suicidal thoughts. He postponed seeking help until his sister prompted him to do so. He had never been to a doctor before, let alone a psychiatrist.

As we see from the dialogue that follows, Anton was struggling with some underlying psychiatric vulnerabilities. Let's first investigate the rules that until now have prevented him from managing the challenges he faced.

> Psychiatrist: I understand that what's brought you here are some suicidal thoughts that are increasingly troubling you?
> Anton: Something like that. My sister was fussing about it, and she talked me into coming.

Here Anton hints at his own ambivalence about seeking help. Could this be something that will yield some useful information?

> Psychiatrist: It sounds like your sister cares about you.... How about you? Are you worried yourself?
> Anton: Well, I'm starting to think that sooner or later I might do something stupid. I can't seem to get out of it. I mean, all the shit that I'm in, but also these, like, horrible thoughts that sort of jump on me.
> Psychiatrist: Yes, suicidal thoughts can be quite scary...and now you have come for help. How does that feel?

The psychiatrist is normalizing and validating the scariness of suicidal thoughts, staying with Anton's ambivalence about seeking help, going slowly, and opening for investigation the ambivalence that has shown up early in the consultation.

> Anton: To be honest, it makes me feel pathetic
>
> Psychiatrist: I can imagine.... You're not alone in that. It takes guts for many people to seek psychiatric help. Do you have a sense of what, for you, feels most pathetic about it?
>
> Anton: I don't see myself as a guy who needs help.
>
> Psychiatrist: You're used to managing on your own?
>
> Anton: That's how I like to be. In the end, it's always up to me...I like that. You never know when other people will mess things up. You've just got to keep on top of things. Just keep doing what you do. I've been low before, and I got through it by working. You just keep working.
>
> Psychiatrist: You're keeping on working, then, rain or shine?
>
> Anton: Yes, I'm working all right. I can work for 18 hours, and then I go home, and then I work again. Work is okay. It's everything else that's going down the drain.
>
> Psychiatrist: Eighteen hours? That's quite a working day! How do you manage to work such long hours?
>
> Anton: I wake up early, sometimes three in the morning, and when I can't sleep again there's nothing else to do except go to work.
>
> Psychiatrist: And even after working such long hours the sleep doesn't come easy?

Anton has laid out one set of rules that he lives by: "In order to be safe, I have to be self-reliant, to manage on my own and not need anyone." The converse would be that it is unsafe to need or to receive help. We may guess that exposing vulnerability or needing help is something he probably associates with weakness. It's hard work, ultimately, that gets you out of trouble.

> Psychiatrist: How about company? Do you make time to see friends now and then? Is there a relationship?
>
> Anton: I go to the bar on Friday nights, but I can't say I have any friends there. We just have beers together. It's easy for me to attract women, real easy, but I don't even care about that now.... I don't know what to do. I just keep feeling more shitty. My sister went for psychiatry a few years back, and I can see it helped her. But me, I don't know what I'm doing here.
>
> Psychiatrist: I see. I'm guessing that you don't know what I'm doing here either?
>
> Anton: (*with a smile*) Yeah—Well, what do you mean?
>
> Psychiatrist: I mean that maybe you're not so used to going to see a doctor.
>
> Anton: I've never been. No offense, but I don't honestly think that anybody can help me. The only reason I've come is that I don't want my daughter to have no dad.

> Psychiatrist: I understand. It doesn't come easy to you to reach out for help. A crisis has had to develop on several fronts at the same time before you felt able to ask for help. That's how hard it is for you to do this. Let's sit with that for a minute.

Here the psychiatrist pauses, not for too long, but long enough to illuminate and validate Anton's extreme discomfort (an acceptance move) and the resulting depth and breadth of this crisis. An imagined consequence of unsafety for relying on others' judgment and help has long been Anton's guiding principle, even when the actual consequences of not seeking help became increasingly serious.

> Psychiatrist: Facing the heartbreaking possibility that your daughter could become fatherless is what it has taken for you to come here, and now you've taken the first step in a new, unknown direction.

The psychiatrist has spent some time bringing into awareness these guiding rules and the effect of them, since the patient's willingness to open up to receive help and to trust the psychiatrist is important to the unfolding of events. The fact that Anton is already trying something new is validated and savored.

> Anton ended up attending appointments over a lengthy period of time, in which a pattern of previous depressive and hypomanic episodes emerged. He chose to trust the psychiatrist's judgment regarding diagnosis and accepted pharmacological treatment for depression for some duration, as well as a longer-term mood stabilizer. He also came to the outpatient care unit every 2 weeks to receive administrative help with paying his bills. After a year, his crisis situation had resolved: his mood was stable, his sleeping pattern was regular, and he had managed to keep his apartment, win shared custody of his daughter, and meet and move in with a woman he truly held dear. The whole of this positive course of events was greatly spurred by the value of being a good father to his daughter. It also built upon an acknowledgment of his previous guiding principles around receiving help and upon a conscious decision to do something different.

Crisis Instigation Through Avoidance

The common response to anything unpleasant in life is to try to avoid it. We respond to outer situations that are dangerous or disagreeable, often quite effectively, by means of emotionally guided behavior. This, in turn, is determined by evolution-shaped learning, model-free learning, and model-based learning. Emotions thus provide the guiding principle for outward responses on the approach–avoid continuum. There are situations, however, in which this outer behavioral repertoire is of very limited use in solving the problem that the inner emotion is signaling, such as when there is nothing we can do to get back a loved one or to escape other types of catastrophes that have already happened. What do we do then?

One common response is to turn our efforts toward trying to escape the inner pain of loss and fear—what has been termed *experiential avoidance* (Hayes et al. 1996, 2011).

Experiential Avoidance: Emotional and Behavioral Avoidance

In crisis, people experience a range of distressing feelings, such as fear, anxiety, anger, shock, distress, grief, and guilt. Unwanted thoughts, memories, images, impulses, and physical sensations add to the burden. All such weighty experiences, whether at the level of body, emotions, or thoughts, need eventually to be integrated. The common, understandable response is to do everything one can to hold these experiences at bay, and sometimes it's functional to first establish a holding capacity—within oneself or with the support of others—before opening up to the pain. In the long run, however, unwillingness to make direct experiential contact with what is going on inside will turn out to be a stick in the wheel of dealing constructively with change and crisis.

Whereas external threats and obstacles can be eliminated or fixed by means of the resourceful human brain, threatening inner experiences cannot be controlled, suppressed, solved, escaped, or avoided. Attempting to do so can amplify them, make them worse. Because the avoidance of inner experience works for a while, as a quick fix, it is an alluring and misleading strategy. All efforts of avoidance, distraction, or repression, regardless of what inner process is being targeted (emotions, memories, tensions, urges), paradoxically result in a long-term increase in the invasiveness and intensity of what is being suppressed from awareness. This is known as the *suppression rebound effect* (Wegner et al. 1987). When we try to eliminate our distressing inner experiences, we do the one thing guaranteed to prolong the agony!

Viewing our involuntary emotional reactions to a crisis as "problems to be solved" not only triggers these attempts to inwardly control or eliminate them—that is, *emotional* avoidance—but also unleashes a wave of outward *behavioral* avoidance strategies intended to avoid entering any situations that may spark negative affect. Emotional and behavioral avoidance are both forms of experiential avoidance—that is, attempts to avoid what is going on inside, be it unwanted feelings, distressing thoughts, or disturbing bodily sensations. As disengagement can be understood as unmindful *doing*, so experiential avoidance can be described as unmindful *being*, because it involves staying out of contact with what is actually going on inside. The two processes of disengagement and avoidance are both based on being unaware of what is going on in the present moment, inwardly and outwardly.

Experiential Avoidance From a Behavior-Analytic Perspective

When we think of the means we commonly use to distance ourselves from what is here to be experienced in the present moment (emotional avoidance)—such as liquor, food, overworking, electronic screens, and so on—we may recognize how these habits are unhelpful. Likewise, we may be aware that avoiding an anxiety-provoking external event by not showing up (behavioral avoidance) often leads to an increased resistance to taking part next time. Why are emotional and behavioral avoidance of inner distress so prevalent when they are clearly not helpful in the longer term? Why do we adhere to these strategies even when we are aware they are not helpful? From a behavior-analytic perspective, these tendencies are propelled by two slightly different mechanisms—rule governance and reinforcement learning—often in conjunction.

Rule Governance in Avoidance

Rule-governed behavior, and the rigid self-instructional sequences it installs, is not only fundamental to disengagement but also one main driver of experiential avoidance. The effectiveness of fixing or avoiding outer problems is interpreted and translated into an approach that applies also to the inner milieu. Intense and distressing inner experiences thereby become specified as a danger to our personal health and well-being that must be eliminated to protect us from harm. In this way, painful internal experiences may trigger reactions in the same way we respond to external threats to health and well-being. The misunderstanding that we can deal with inner distress the same way we deal with outer problems is supported by the short-term reward of transitory relief that comes with avoidance. However, although we can avoid or control a fear-provoking external stimulus, we cannot in the long term avoid inner fear. In general, it is more advantageous to pay attention to inner experiences and either learn what they are trying to convey or investigate their validity. Therefore, outer and inner problems cannot be approached with the same type of solutions—yet that is exactly what we often try to do. In ACT, this is known as the *unworkable change agenda*. Many of our waking hours are spent trying to control or eliminate inner distress. Experiential avoidance consumes not only time but also a lot of energy and comes in many guises. Each of us has ones we prefer.

Because of the ease with which language can produce psychological rigidity in following rules and hence cause suffering, people easily fall into organized patterns of rule-governed behavior that enable them to escape or control painful thoughts, emotions, and memories. In contemporary society, one widespread message is that the way to be healthy is to rid oneself of anything unpleasant, unwanted, or untoward. In reality, however, we become healthier, wiser, and steadier through receiving and allowing whatever experience may arise. Another widely cultivated belief is that "normal" people do not have significant problems with emotional discomfort or when confronted with a crisis; they are "strong enough" to simply overpower their emotional pain by directly controlling or eliminating it. This belief places the average person at almost continuous risk of suffering because attempts to control, eliminate, or suppress emotional discomfort produce exactly the result one is trying avoid—making the distress feel even more invasive and uncontrollable.

Reinforcement Through Rule Governance: Short-Term Versus Long-Term Consequences

Experiential avoidance relies on strategies linked to short-term consequences rather than long-term goals. The immediate but temporary alleviation of distress that we obtain will affect our choices through negative reinforcement. If the mode of distraction consists of further short-term rewards—such as food, shopping, or computer games—we will simultaneously be influenced by short-term rewards. If, for example, instead of experiencing our feeling of loneliness and need for connection, we fill the void with an extra piece of cake, we obtain a momentary distraction and relief from the pain of loneliness (negative reinforcement); if we are timid, we also evade the discomfort of reaching out for company (negative reinforcement); and we get a temporary rush from the sweet taste of the cake (positive reinforcement). The long-term effects of prolonged loneliness do not then influence our choices as strongly as these short-term consequences.

Another long-term effect is that the distress of isolation will eventually come back in a stronger and sometimes more confusing package, which may prompt us to try even harder to get rid of our inner affliction by pursuing the short-term reward of emotional pain relief. This spiral of seeking distraction from pain may escalate into a situation with which we are unable to deal. We may possibly then reach out for professional help, or we may consider more drastic and dangerous strategies to avoid our inner pain—such as suicide.

As we explore in depth in Chapter 7, one way to counteract the influence of the cycle of short-term rewards is to remind ourselves of our long-term purposes and values. Particularly in crisis situations, it is pivotal to understand and to be highly alert to the reinforcing effects that short-term outcomes have on our choices.

Emotional Avoidance

States of negative emotion are the most common kind of private experience that we try to avoid. The main reason we avoid experiencing certain kinds of thoughts and memories is that contacting those inner experiences will directly give rise to intense negative emotions.

Emotional avoidance is the unwillingness to make contact with distressing, unwanted emotions; this term refers to *anything* that is used as a means to avoid inner experiences (Figure 2–2). We can *distract* ourselves from feeling (by binge-watching miniseries or the news, working long hours, or immersing ourselves in social media and surfing the internet). We can use *substances* (food, alcohol, drugs, tobacco, numbing types of medications). The common use of alcohol and drugs to regulate uncomfortable feelings is an excellent example of how short-term consequences may guide behavior at the expense of long-term ones; the choice to prioritize bringing relief to the moment not only causes physiological imbalance the next day but also commonly aggravates the situation in general. We can attempt to *suppress* (push down the feelings that are there) or *ignore* (be oblivious of our bodily and emotional responses). We can turn to *risky activities* (seeking out dangerous situations, engaging in incautious sex, gambling, or fast driving) that evoke even stronger urgent emotions that drown out the underlying ones. We can contemplate *suicide*, the ultimate solution to put an end to a devastating inner experience or crisis situation that appears *inescapable, interminable*, and experientially *intolerable*—the three "I"s (Chiles et al. 2018). A severe long-term challenge or an instantaneous desolating loss can bring a person to the brink of what they believe they can endure. Other times, the outer situation may be less challenging yet exceed the person's present capacity for acceptance, engagement with their values, and problem-solving.

There is also a fourth "I": an overwhelming sense of *isolation* and being on your own in carrying extreme internal and external hardship. This sense of being cut off from the rest of humanity is a cardinal feature of a

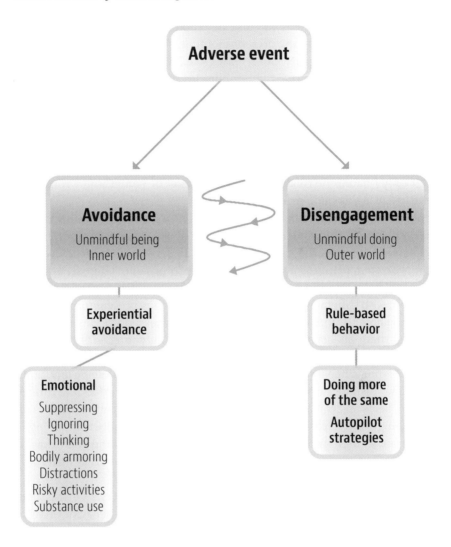

Figure 2–2.   Crisis instigation through emotional avoidance.

suicidal crisis, something we return to in Chapter 6, "Acceptance and Self-Compassion." For those who experienced trauma and abuse during childhood, suicidality can be understood as a way to deal with feelings of shame and self-disgust by punishing themselves. In sum, suicidality can be seen as a drastic pathway to avoiding intense suffering. The good news is that a suicidal crisis can be tackled with the same crisis integration tools as can other types of crises.

More subtle processes can also be employed in avoiding the experience of what is here in the present moment, such as tensing our muscles to brace ourselves against our feelings (e.g., when we tighten our throat, chest, or belly). Just as we tighten muscles in response to physical pain, we can tense around emotional pain and somatic distress. With time, these tensions may become long-held patterns of *bodily armoring*. Such processes can be so familiar and unobtrusive that they go unnoticed. Another avoidance strategy involves *thinking*: dwelling on past experiences, planning for or worrying about the future, or blaming others or yourself ("If only I had done this or that"; "There must be something wrong with me because this happened").

It is worth pausing here to acknowledge the perhaps counterintuitive feel of some of this. One might imagine that staying present to the inner effects of the instigating circumstances of a crisis would equate to dwelling on, worrying, blaming, and trying to figure things out. There is, however, a subtle but profound distinction between "thinking about" and "staying present with" (meta-awareness) experiences. Staying present to experiences means allowing and receiving them with awareness, observing them, and letting them be just as they are. There is nothing wrong with thinking—when investigating the cause of suffering or when problem-solving, for example—but it needs to alternate with attending to and allowing emotions. One may also be surprised to learn that worrying, uncomfortable though it may be, is an avoidance strategy; the emotions to which the worry is responding—often fear—may be apprehended as much more frightening to confront, at least initially. In a similar way, as disheartening and exhausting as self-blame is, it facilitates emotional avoidance of other unsettling and chaotic experiences triggered by the crisis events.

Because substance abuse is such a prevalent factor in crisis instigation, let us spell out the mechanisms underlying it from a behavior-analytic perspective. Although substances sometimes are used to experience joy and elation, the more common and problematic use of substances is in service of avoiding difficult inner experiences. Even when substances are initially used recreationally, the behavior is positively reinforced and, after extensive indulgence over time, becomes a means of emotional avoidance of withdrawal symptoms and craving. Like all avoidance strategies, the use of substances provides relief from anguish on a short-term basis and thus is negatively reinforced.

In this way, substance use disorders can be construed as a loop of crisis instigation with four domains of likely problems. The first concerns how the patient relates to uncomfortable experiences. Can they tolerate distress, or do they tend to avoid it? Second, how does the patient relate to anxieties relating to withdrawal symptoms? When one fears such after effects, it is an easy step to keep using the substance in order to avoid them. And what about craving—the strong urge to keep using the substance that has previously provided such rewarding experiences? Can the patient stay present to a wave of craving without being compelled to act on it? Third, how has the substance impacted the patient's social identity? Do they use substances to overcome shyness or social anxiety or to minimize self-critical thoughts during social interaction? Do most of their social interactions now involve the use of substances? Whereas the aforementioned three domains pertain to negatively reinforced emotional avoidance, the fourth concerns the degree to which substance abuse has caused a loss of values and engagement. Does the patient spend most of their spare time drinking, such that they no longer have any sense of meaningful sober activity? If they have lost their family, friends, and work because of their addiction, they may have forgotten their values altogether, their main pursuit having narrowed down to obtaining the next high. An assessment of the patient's specific tendencies in these four aspects will create a foundation for designing an appropriate program of crisis integration.

Behavioral Avoidance

Behavioral avoidance is an active retreat from situations, events, or interactions that could trigger unpleasant, unwanted inner experiences (Figure 2–3). A common way to practice behavioral avoidance is to keep away from situations that might produce negative emotions. Behavioral avoidance is one major reason why patients spiral into crisis and why they eventually seek professional help. It is closely related to rule-following in that rules may initially be formulated for the sake of avoiding discomfort, but behavioral avoidance involves something else too, as we discuss later. It may take the form of well-organized problem-solving and yet ultimately be destructive because this activity is designed mainly to reduce emotional distress.

Emotional avoidance is a secret affliction because no one can see you avoiding your own experiences. *Behavioral avoidance*, on the other hand, entails avoiding participation in key areas of life, and this directly leads to functional decline. Functional decline in turn is associated with a host of further negative social consequences that may trigger even more negative states of emotion. The short-term consequence of behavioral avoidance is escape from the immediate discomfort of painful moments and situations. In the vocabulary of behavioral psychology, actions chosen to avoid short-term discomfort are governed by negative reinforcement. The obvi-

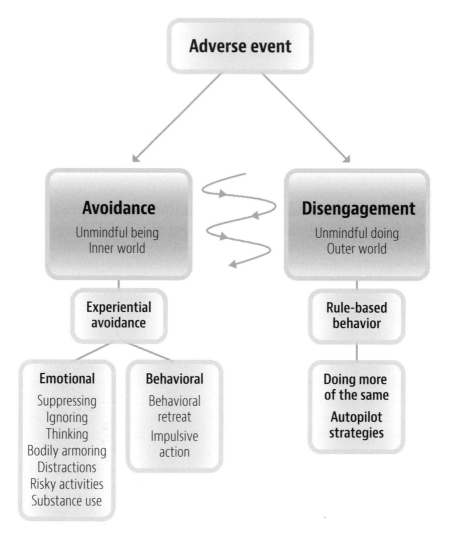

Figure 2–3.   Crisis instigation through behavioral avoidance.

ous long-term consequences consecutively involve passivity, self-isolation, loss of social connectedness, and declining motivation and skill to perform necessary daily tasks—a common presentation in psychiatric practice and certainly fertile ground for chronic distress and crises. Our core premise is that experiential avoidance, together with rule-following, is responsible for most of people's suffering in the realm of inner experiences generally and of personal crisis specifically.

In some unfortunate cases, behavioral avoidance leads to another type of behavioral response: that of not acting at all. Behavioral avoidance tends to expand into progressively larger areas of life, culminating eventually in the response of *behavioral retreat*. Behavioral retreat may also include ignoring facts, even when they are right before your eyes, and abstaining from responding to a situation that obviously needs to be addressed. The negative reinforcement loop associated with non-action relies on the short-term relief of distress, at the price of long-term functional decline and increasing despair. When the inner container becomes overloaded with emotional charge, *impulsive action* can be another short-term solution to escape the pressing situation. Impulsive behaviors such as acting out or emotional venting can be an effective quick fix, but in the long run they poison the well of social connectedness. Let us explore with a clinical example how emotional and behavioral avoidance may instigate a long-standing crisis.

For most of us, the acute distress of a catastrophe wanes with time. Waves of excruciating pain may continue to arise, possibly for as long as we live, but if we allow and receive them, they will subside again. We can then engage in what needs to be dealt with, one day at a time, while gradually integrating what has happened. For some people, however, persistent and debilitating suffering continues for years and years; it may even deepen over time through the mechanisms of experiential avoidance, as happened for Kai.

Kai: Clinical Dialogue on Crisis Instigation With Experiential Avoidance at a Late Stage

Kai is 35 years of age, single, living at home with his parents, and has no income of his own. He didn't show up for his scheduled appointment at the psychiatric outpatient clinic a month ago, but he has come today to the crisis intervention unit associated with his community mental health center. He sits and shakes, making very little eye contact. It is difficult to imagine, but 7 years ago he was a high-functioning individual. He lived with his girlfriend of several years, ran his own restaurant, and had a nice circle of friends and acquaintances. However, when he was about to move his restaurant to a new location, he discovered that his business partner had defrauded him. He was left deeply in debt, and eventually his business went bankrupt. He sued his partner and would probably have won the case, but he became severely anxious and panic-stricken and asked his lawyer to withdraw his claim.

From then on, the crisis spiraled downward. Kai ruminated about what had happened, tying his mind in a knot trying to make sense of the situation, shifting back and forth between blaming his business partner and blaming himself. He lost sleep, was highly irritable, and suffered bouts of depression, anxiety, and panic. His relationship with his girlfriend steadily deteriorated because of his emotional problems, and she eventually left him for another man she had met at work. After he filed for bankruptcy, Kai was forced to sell his restaurant at a fraction of what it was worth. He lost his entire life savings, could no longer pay his own living costs, and moved back in with his parents. With the passing of time, he became more isolated and lost contact with his friends, spending most of his days alone in his room. He was rarely eating meals with his parents and had no routines of sleep and mealtimes.

Kai had taken part in a behavioral activation group at the mental health center but had dropped out after just a few group sessions. He had also tried several types of antidepressant medication and a repetitive transcranial magnetic stimulation (rTMS) treatment without lasting success.

Psychiatrist: This is the first time you and I have met, but I did have a chance to go over your chart, so we have a bit of a head start.

Kai: Okay.

Psychiatrist: How are you feeling today?

Kai: Lousy. I stopped taking the new antidepressant they prescribed for me. It didn't seem to work at all.

Psychiatrist: I see. When you say it didn't work, what do you have in mind?

Kai: I tried it for a few months. I even tried TMS. I thought initially that I was getting better, but no, there was no change really. I just feel like my life is over. Nothing seems to help. I feel just as bad as ever.

Psychiatrist: I'm sorry to hear that. When you feel bad, and you're at home, what does that look like? If I were a fly on the wall, what would I see you doing or not doing?

Kai: (*silence*) I don't know. As soon as I think about doing something—going out or something—I get so scared that I don't know what to do. So I make an excuse not to go. My friends don't call me anymore because they know I'll never show up. I don't understand what's wrong with me, even though I've tried to figure it out. I didn't use to feel this way. I used to be able to deal with stuff, you know, but now it's like I can't handle anything.

Psychiatrist: So when you get this intense fear or anxiety and you've decided to stay at home instead of doing whatever you were supposed to do, what happens next?

Kai: I just get really down and hopeless and go to my room and try to put it out of my mind. But instead, I'm, like, reliving everything that's happened, all these failures and losses. I try to make sense of it all. Like, what I did or didn't do and why. The low point was when Judy, my girlfriend, met another guy at work and moved in with him. That really hurt. Before all this shit happened, we were planning on getting married. I blame myself for letting her down. I know it's not good for me to hide away, but it's the only way I can feel a bit less panicked. I don't know what else to do. I'm just not the same person I used to be. (*Looks down, holding his arms tightly round his body.*)

> I need to get back to the person I was, but there doesn't seem to be anything to help me do that.
>
> Psychiatrist: It sounds like when you're about to do something, maybe get out of the house or go and do something around town, this sense of fear and anxiety shows up and blocks you from doing that. And you have no idea why all of this is happening, even though you've analyzed it a lot. I'm guessing you've probably analyzed it from every possible angle, but that doesn't seem to be getting you anywhere.

It is good, certainly, to analyze a situation in order to learn from mistakes, but when this is done in excess—in the form of rumination—and without balancing such thinking with staying present to your inner experiences as they are, the going over and over it in your head may be understood as emotional avoidance. Such rumination has caused Kai's fear and stress to come back in magnified and different forms—an example of the suppression rebound effect.

> Kai: (*silence*) I'm scared I will always be this way. This is no life, being scared all the time, having no friends, no job, no future. It's hopeless. (*Tears up and rocks back and forth.*) I couldn't even complete the group therapy thing they said would help me. How am I ever going to feel better? (*quietly*) It's all my fault.
>
> Psychiatrist: It's all your fault?
>
> Kai: Yes, I let all this happen, and I lost everything.
>
> Psychiatrist: "All this"?
>
> Kai: I was so stupid that I let myself be cheated in the first place; I didn't check up on what my partner was doing. When I sued him for the money I'd lost, I realized I would never be able to handle the pressure of going to court. So I chickened out and let him get away with it. I still can't understand why I did that. Everything in my life has gone downhill since then.

Kai's withdrawal of his legal case was a move of *behavioral* avoidance, as are his ongoing decisions to stay at home whenever his anxiety mounted as he began to step out the door. His avoidance strategies, both emotional and behavioral, are negatively reinforced when they release him from short-term discomfort. The long-term consequences are reduced functionality and participation in life, which naturally give rise to further difficulties, exacerbating this prolonged crisis situation.

> Psychiatrist: When you say that everything has gone downhill since that awful moment when you got cheated, what does "going downhill" look like?
>
> Kai: I don't do anything anymore. I'm nervous about every little thing. Just thinking of taking the bus somewhere gets me panicking. In the

group I went to they told us to "do things anyway," even when you feel down or nervous. But no one understands. No one understands what it's like to be afraid all the time. The only way to escape that is to stay in my room and try to sleep if I can.

Psychiatrist: Could you give me an example of a recent time when you tried to go out of the house, so I can get a sense of how this works?

Kai: Okay…. This one's kind of typical. I told my mom that I'd go to the drugstore and pick up some medicines her doctor had prescribed for her because she had the flu or something and didn't feel good. I got dressed and was ready to go, but each time I tried to open the front door, I just couldn't do it. I felt so scared. I was dizzy, shaking, couldn't think straight. My legs felt so weak, I thought I might pass out. So I went back to my room. My mom didn't know I hadn't gone and came up to my room to ask me where her medicines were. I told her I hadn't gone. I felt so bad because she had to get dressed and go get them.

Psychiatrist: (*after a pause*) Can you tell me what happened when you went to your room? I mean, before your mom showed up?

Kai: What I felt was relief. I felt better. My fear gets better when I go to my room, at least for a while. Then I start to think about all the things that have happened and what's wrong with me.

The short-term consequence of *relief* that Kai gets from retreating into his room provides negative reinforcement of the very same behavior.

Psychiatrist: So the fear comes back after a while, even when you're alone in your room?

Kai: Yeah, it does, but it is not a full-fledged panic-type fear like the kind I get when I think about going out somewhere, or riding on a bus, or going to an appointment or something like that.

Psychiatrist: If now you think over the years since all of this began, and about the strategies you've been using to keep your anxiety and fear under control—things like thinking about what you did wrong, not leaving your house, trying to sleep as much as you can, avoiding social activities with your friends, staying in your room a lot—would you say your fear has gotten better over the years, or has it gotten worse?

Kai: It's worse. Way worse. I have no life right now.

Psychiatrist: Well, you've been through the ringer, Kai. Being cheated by someone you trusted, having your business ruined, losing what sounds like the love of your life, and having to deal with all those high-stress legal and financial issues. That would be a big drain on anyone. A clear 10 on the stress scale is hard to bounce back from.

Kai: I haven't bounced back at all. I think almost anyone would have somehow started their life again, but not me.

In a continuous effort to control the magnitude of his emotional experience, Kai has developed a pattern of withdrawing from any demand that might trigger more distress. Backing out of situations that he fears rather than moving forward and through the anxiety of taking part in life again is a classic feature of behavioral avoidance and illustrates how it can become so self-destructive. In Chapter 7 we see how the crisis integration process unfolds for Kai.

Moment-to-Moment Choices Made in Difficult Circumstances

We have seen that the real problem when dealing with challenges is the combination of avoiding our inner experiences and acting according to previously learned rules and strategies. This is not an aberration but, rather, as we have seen in this chapter and continue to explore, a quite natural consequence of the human brain's learning mechanisms, which in their different ways lead to flexibility, stability, and in crisis instigation even rigidity. The ACT approach to crisis involves addressing these learning systems. What determines whether the state of crisis continues and deepens is the way we respond to the change that's happened: whether we turn away from what life has given us to experience, comprehend, and integrate and continue to rely on insidious habits when choosing our actions, or explore unfamiliar terrains, both inside and outside. The extent to which we are willing to be flexible and to be altered by the changed reality, taking life one moment at a time, is what in the end will determine the amount of suffering we will undergo. The next chapter gives an overview of how these processes of crisis instigation can be addressed in clinical practice.

References

Carlsson K, Petrovic P, Skare S, et al: Tickling expectations: neural processing in anticipation of a sensory stimulus. J Cogn Neurosci 12(4):691–703, 2000 10936920

Carlsson K, Petersson KM, Lundqvist D, et al: Fear and the amygdala: manipulation of awareness generates differential cerebral responses to phobic and fear-relevant (but nonfeared) stimuli. Emotion 4(4):340–353, 2004 15571433

Chiles J, Strosahl K, Roberts L: Clinical Manual for Assessment and Treatment of Suicidal Patients, 2nd Edition. Washington, DC, American Psychiatric Association Publishing, 2018

Damasio AR: The Feeling of What Happens: Body and Emotion in the Making of Consciousness. Orlando, FL, Harcourt Brace, 1999

Dolan RJ: Emotion, cognition, and behavior. Science 298(5596):1191–1194, 2002 12424363

Frith C: Making Up the Mind: How the Brain Creates Our Mental World. Malden, MA, Blackwell Publishing, 2007, pp 10–45

Frith C: The neural basis of consciousness. Psychol Med 51(4):550–562, 2021 31481140

Frith C, Dolan RJ: Brain mechanisms associated with top-down processes in perception. Philos Trans R Soc Lond B Biol Sci 352(1358):1221–1230, 1997 9304688

Goubert DP, Törneke N, Purssey R, et al: Learning Acceptance and Commitment Therapy: The Essential Guide to the Process and Practice of Mindful Psychiatry. Washington, DC, American Psychiatric Association Publishing, 2020

Hayes SC, Wilson KG, Gifford EV, et al: Experimental avoidance and behavioral disorders: a functional dimensional approach to diagnosis and treatment. J Consult Clin Psychol 64(6):1152–1168, 1996 8991302

Hayes SC, Barnes-Holmes D, Roche B (eds): Relational Frame Theory: A Post-Skinnerian Account of Human Language and Cognition. New York, Springer, 2001

Hayes SC, Strosahl KD, Wilson KG: Acceptance and Commitment Therapy, 2nd Edition: The Process and Practice of Mindful Change. New York, Guilford, 2011

Huys QJM, Cruickshank A, Series P: Reward-based learning, model-based and model-free, in Encyclopedia of Computational Neuroscience. Edited by Jaeger DJ, Jung R. New York, Springer New York, 2014, pp 1–10

Kahneman D: Thinking, Fast and Slow. New York, Farrar, Straus, & Giroux, 2011

LeDoux J: The Emotional Brain: The Mysterious Underpinnings of Emotional Life. New York, Simon & Schuster, 1998

Lindeblad BN: Closed fist, open palm, in I May Be Wrong: And Other Wisdoms From Life as a Forest Monk. London, Bloomsbury, 2022, pp 117–120

McClure SM, Laibson DI, Loewenstein G, et al: Separate neural systems value immediate and delayed monetary rewards. Science 306(5695):503–507, 2004 15486304

Nowak MA, Tarnita CE, Wilson EO: The evolution of eusociality. Nature 466(7310):1057–1062, 2010 20740005

Öhman A, Carlsson K, Lundqvist D, et al: On the unconscious subcortical origin of human fear. Physiol Behav 92(1–2):180–185, 2007 17599366

Schultz W: Behavioral theories and the neurophysiology of reward. Annu Rev Psychol 57:87–115, 2006 16318590

Vatansever D, Menon DK, Stamatakis EA: Default mode contributions to automated information processing. Proc Natl Acad Sci USA 114(48):12821–12826, 2017 29078345

Villatte M, Villatte JL, Hayes SC: Mastering the Clinical Conversation: Language as Intervention. New York, Guilford, 2019

Wegner DM, Schneider DJ, Carter SR 3rd, et al: Paradoxical effects of thought suppression. J Pers Soc Psychol 53(1):5–13, 1987 3612492

3

The ACT Model of Crisis Integration

In Zen there are only two things: you sit and you sweep the garden. It doesn't matter how big the garden is.

—Oda Sesso*

Crisis Integration With Acceptance, Mindfulness, and Engagement

When a serious life event or catastrophe is pushing us to the limit of what we can accommodate psychologically, we need some guiding principles we can keep coming back to. When the world as we knew it has been shattered, when we can no longer distinguish up from down, we need simple and timeless counsel we can depend on. Our premise in this book is that we will eventually ride through anything life throws at us as long as we hold on to the three processes of acceptance, mindfulness, and engagement.

These processes provide not merely a starting point or an endpoint but the basis from which, in the turmoil of crisis, we may begin again in each and every moment. They provide a solid foundation that will always be there to launch from and to fall back upon. It usually doesn't matter much which of the three processes we choose to employ in any given moment of a crisis. All three will offer insight, compassion, healing, and rest and will reveal new strategies to explore.

---

* From Snyder 1980.

This chapter draws on a series of dialogues to provide an overview of the ACT model of crisis integration. In the case studies of the previous chapter, we were primarily interested in identifying the specific psychological processes that contribute to crisis *instigation*. Here we'll pick up one of these clinical narratives and introduce another to illustrate what the processes of crisis *integration* may look like in practice. Our goal is to better acquaint readers with the model as a whole before we dive deeper, in subsequent chapters, into the nuances of theory and practice for each of the three core processes—acceptance, mindfulness, and engagement—that facilitate crisis integration.

Much of what the psychiatrist does in the dialogues that follow models ways in which these processes can be applied. This modeling aims to inspire patients to emulate what they have experienced in a session so that they can then apply the same principles in their lives afterward. However, although it is easy to talk the talk of acceptance, mindfulness, and engagement, it can be difficult to walk the walk in practice, particularly in the heat of a crisis. The psychiatrist may encounter features in a crisis reaction that trigger an internal negative judgment of a patient, which makes it hard to model acceptance. When that happens, it is important to recognize that psychiatrists are human beings as well, and do have blind spots. The psychiatrist can turn again to acceptance—this time, acceptance of their own inner reactions, whether they be judgments, impatience, or disapproval. Paying close attention to our own reactions in the moment will reveal valuable information about what we need to learn in order to expand our capacity for acceptance and compassion. This journey of discovery will prove to be a lifetime endeavor for anyone who chooses to travel it, because there is no limit to the amount of acceptance, mindfulness, and engagement we can bring into the world.

There's also certainly not just one way to model and guide patients toward acceptance, mindfulness, and engagement during a clinical session; there are as many ways as there are psychiatrists and patients. As long as the psychiatrist remembers to employ for themselves the very principles they advocate for patients, they will be able to find their own way of applying these processes in the midst of a clinical crisis.

Acceptance

Acceptance can be thought of functionally as the opposite of avoidance. Instead of trying to change or grapple with painful inner experiences, we allow what is there to be there. Instead of turning away from distress, we lean in and listen to what is happening inside. Instead of overidentifying

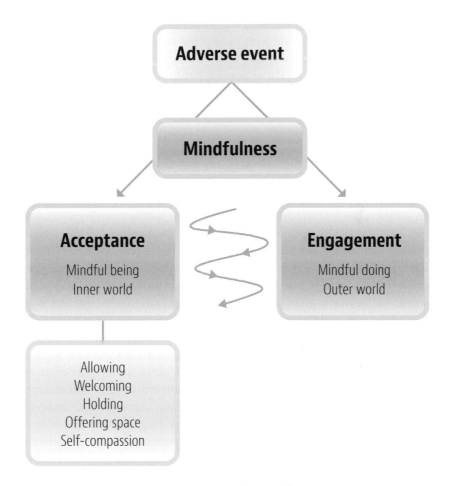

Figure 3–1.   Crisis integration through acceptance.

with immediate experience and letting it define who we are in that moment, we disidentify from the experience and hold it in kindness and affection (Figure 3–1).

Certain misconceptions about acceptance may be held by both patients and psychiatrists. First, we do not practice acceptance with the aim that the emotional pain will disappear. It is impossible to know what will happen if we do nothing but remain accepting, give the pain some air, and be open to the natural evolution of uncontested inner experience. The pain may increase or decrease in intensity, or it may not change at all. This is why acceptance requires an outlook of curiosity on the part of both patient and psychiatrist. Second, acceptance does not mean resigning oneself to suffering or giving up because we've been defeated by the overwhelming force of our inner experiences. Patients will sometimes ask the rhetorical question, "Do you mean I should just give up and let the suffering go on?" All acceptance does is allow us to give up on trying to control what we cannot change. We do not have to like what is happening inside in order to practice acceptance. The stance of being nonjudgmental prevents us from making things worse. What we then are left with is the original pain that entered our life, without the additional layer of suffering related to non-acceptance. Acceptance is a powerful emotion regulation strategy in its own right and should be a key part of the toolkit of any psychiatrist who works with patients in crisis. Third, acceptance in an ongoing injurious situation, such as an abusive relationship, definitely does not mean accepting the abuse itself, or even the relationship. Acceptance here means opening up to and fully knowing the inner desolation and the unmet need for safety, whereafter the logical next step will be to seek protection from the abuse. Fourth, acceptance is sometimes misconceived as implying passivity and non-action. To the contrary, the time and energy spent on avoiding inner experiences will be free to apply toward actions in pursuit of what matters to us.

Dictionaries define *acceptance* as "general agreement that something is satisfactory or right" or "agreement to a plan or suggestion" (Cambridge University Press 2022; Macmillan 2022). In ACT, acceptance is not about agreeing; it's about knowing and caring for the inner pain that arises in response to outer adversity. Acceptance also entails letting go of resistance to knowing the outer reality as it is—in other words, moving from unawareness or denial to seeing clearly what's going on. From this new position of clarity, we can more effectively engage with injustices around us, with the intent of bringing about change: "This is what's happening. What can I do about it?" Through commitment to values of environmental protection, peace, equity, inclusion, diversity, and social justice, we can find the motivation to undertake and support initiatives, local or worldwide, that serve these timeless values.

Finally, when the outer situation can't be changed, acceptance does include acknowledging and embracing the way things are. Caution is needed here, however. The demand to accept a grim situation or a fundamental loss can feel like an extra burden upon an already heavy soul. Patients are likely to respond with, "Yeah, yeah, 'Accept what is'—that's easy to say! I don't want it to be this way. I can imagine that eventually I'll tolerate it, but don't ask me to accept it!" and they're right, because this demand overlooks some crucial steps. David, whom we met in Chapter 2 ("The ACT Model of Crisis Instigation"), had recently injured his spinal cord. For him, "acceptance of what is" needed to start with the inner experiences, with the desperation of "not wanting it to be this way" (avoidance) and the underlying somatic and emotional responses to unmet needs and values. Then and only then can he close in on accepting the outer situation as changed. If David were to sidestep his inner distress and directly aim to accept the excruciating new situation, he would be doing the exact opposite of accepting. He'd be striving to ignore, suppress, reason with, or completely escape his inner reality. Sidestepping inner responses when working on acceptance is so prevalent, among both patients and psychiatrists, that we want to call attention to this phenomenon by giving it a name: "the acceptance fallacy."

Upon meeting David, one might feel eager to encourage him to take part in his rehabilitation, his obvious task at hand, or at least to limit his impulsive and self-defeating behavior by reasoning with him. However, David probably already knows all the good reasons for rehab work, and he still isn't coming to do it. Thus, one needs to begin by uncovering his reasons for not showing up—and for his building an even greater disconnect from his life, such as contemplating divorce. The psychiatrist needs to get closer to what David is experiencing and bring awareness and acceptance to some of the pain he is trying to avoid. The old principle of "connect before correct" is valid, and acceptance is a reliable tool to make connection happen—that is, to get patients to feel they are being heard, that their psychic pain is recognized and understood.

In a clinical situation, we can model acceptance through reflecting, validating, and dignifying the inner experiences with which a patient is wrestling. The psychiatrist will want the patient to know that such experiences are common and are encountered by others in similar situations. This approach not only creates a trusting connection between psychiatrist and patient but also nurtures the compassionate and accepting attitude we would like to see in the patient. Acceptance can be conveyed overtly, by voicing it in words, and silently, in the ways the psychiatrist listens to the patient or maintains eye contact during difficult moments in the clinical conversation.

David's psychiatrist first encountered his irritability, but what first meets the eye is generally only the tip of the iceberg. Beneath David's irritability, other substantial experiences awaited discovery. Once that irritability had been given attention and been allowed to stay in the room, one level of experience after another was revealed: David's sense of loneliness connected to a need for understanding; his hopelessness, despair, and worthlessness; and his fear of being unlovable and abandoned. Such unpacking of layers of experience is characteristic of clinical interviewing that is curious in nature and nonjudgmental and accepting in tone. The further the psychiatrist went in listening to successive levels of David's feelings, the more fundamental were the needs and values exposed.

It can be effective to touch on each experience the patient expresses, reflecting back what is said in a completely accepting way. In David's case, if the psychiatrist had jumped ahead with "I guess you're scared of losing love," David would probably not have felt understood to the degree he did when every level of experience was allowed to surface by itself. This doesn't mean the psychiatrist has to reflect back every single experience the patient brings up. If the connection and trust are there, the psychiatrist can choose to listen silently to some of what the patient presents and to reflect out loud others of their feelings and needs. As we pick up on the session with David at the point where we left off in Chapter 2, we see the importance of slowing the pace. When experiences that have previously been avoided are gently contacted, they can be understood in a different way.

David: Clinical Dialogue on Acceptance

> David: I can't bear the thought of looking into her eyes and seeing that she's lost her affection for me.
>
> Psychiatrist: Imagining your wife's love waning, fearing that that will happen, that whole thing—could we stay with that for a little while?
>
> David: What do you mean, "stay with it"?
>
> Psychiatrist: I mean spending some time with those feelings. The fear of the possibility of losing love, and the pain that comes with that.
>
> David: That sounds really hard.
>
> Psychiatrist: I know. The idea is to see if we might offer some company to these feelings of fear and pain. Maybe even bring in a kind of caring for them, as if you were holding the fear and the pain in a caring pair of arms, if that makes sense to you.

Here the psychiatrist is touching on two slightly different moves in acceptance: *feeling* the pain versus *receiving* the pain with equanimity and care. There's a subtle difference that we explore later in this chapter and in the chapters that follow. David, meanwhile, has burst into tears.

> Psychiatrist: Yes. The pain…stay with it…and, good, stay in touch with it a bit longer if you can…

The psychiatrist could, of course, reassure David that his wife is showing no sign of walking out on him, that in fact quite the opposite is true, or she could encourage him not to think, right now, about that possible future scenario coming to pass. However, in acceptance we are curious about what is actually going on rather than what we would like to see happen in the patient. When emotions are simply allowed to be and the patient gets to know them, they will exert less influence on behavioral choices. This opens up the possibility that experiencing emotional pain and choosing one's actions can become separate psychological processes. Moreover, acceptance encourages the patient to adopt a caring stance toward their aching feelings. The psychiatrist therefore encourages the patient to spend some time with the painful feelings that are coming up and models an accepting and compassionate witnessing stance. By providing positive feedback that this is where the patient needs to be for a while, the psychiatrist sets up a situation in which the patient can learn what "staying with it" may feel like.

> David: It's just too much! I can't stand it.
> Psychiatrist: (*quietly*) I know. Just stay a little longer, allowing it to be here with you. And breathe with it.
> David: (*more tears*)
> Psychiatrist: Good work.
> David: I can't keep it in! I'm going to burst.

By "it," David may be referring to the emotions, or to the somatic sensations related to those feelings, that have been activated in his predicament. These will probably have increased in strength through his holding them compressed inside him. What he's saying here could be interpreted as a request to back off, which the psychiatrist could have done for a little while. At times, though, it can be fruitful to nudge the patient to feel a bit more of what is there to be experienced. Whenever patients try to avoid experiencing something, they will also try to get the listener to back off in order to facilitate that avoidance. The psychiatrist's guidance of the patient to allow instead of avoid will, of course, need to be gentle and respectful.

One effect of suppressing emotions can be likened to what happens in a pressure cooker. Suppressing is like putting a lid on the emotions; they intensify and become even scarier. The moment we move from avoidance to acceptance—from suppression to opening up—a well of acute discomfort may arise. Let's see how acceptance processes can, in a very concrete way, continue to offer space to David's "fear of losing love."

> Psychiatrist: Ah, the feelings need space. How much space would you say?
> David: No idea.
> Psychiatrist: Would they fill this room? Could you imagine a pair of arms holding it all and extending as wide as this room?
> David: It would need more than that.
> Psychiatrist: Certainly. Imagine all the space the feelings need, the arms extending far out to encompass the plains, the valleys, the waters, and the mountains of our Earth.

David: It's still not enough.

Psychiatrist: All right, we can include the whole vast sky.

David: Now we're getting close. (*with an ironic little laugh*)

Psychiatrist: Good. Stay with it. Offer space to the fear, the despair, the pain. Imagine them having *all* the space they need, being held in the tender arms of earth and sky, expanding as much as they need. At the same time, we're offering company to these feelings. And, again, breathe…

David: (*after a little while*) It's starting to feel a bit lighter, but now what? Nothing has changed! I'm still here with these useless legs.

Psychiatrist: I want to suggest that we just stay for a little while with that lighter feeling and give that some time and space. We can talk about the other things in due course, but for now, just stay with the change in what you're feeling.

When David's thoughts started wandering off to something else, the psychiatrist could have gone with him and reflected his new thoughts, but on this occasion she chose to encourage him to stay with the experiences that had come up. David described these feelings in terms of somatic sensations; to support an open, curious exploration of what is actually there to be known, the psychiatrist sustains this descriptive mode.

David: Okay.

Psychiatrist: Might you be able to say a bit more about this lighter feeling? To describe what it feels like? Take your time, there's no rush.

David: Well, my chest feels a bit less dense, as if I can breathe more easily.

Psychiatrist: Your chest feels a bit less dense…. Anything else?

David: A bit less thick around my head. Less tense, maybe? This sounds just weird.

Psychiatrist: Weird is fine. Let's stay a little longer with that feeling of "less tense" around your head.

David: It's like I had clamps around my skull, and they've loosened their grip a little.

Psychiatrist: That sounds like a nice change. Just stay with it, for as long as you like.

David: (*after some time*) Wow, I'm really tired now!

Psychiatrist: Okay, this seems like a good point at which to stop. You've done something really important today. You've allowed space for some of your anguish instead of pushing it down. Let's take one thing at a time. You're in the midst of a major crisis in your life. It's a situation that demands lots of learning, probably way more new learning than you've had to do since you were a kid. It will inevitably take time to take this all in and figure out how to move forward. I would suggest that you postpone making any major life decisions—such as whether to stay in or leave your marriage—for the time being. There will be plenty of time to figure such things out once you get your sails adjusted to this new direction your life is taking. Right now, just rest for a while. I'll be back tomorrow to see how you're doing.

Here, the psychiatrist has provided a short explanation of what they have been doing, making the process of acceptance explicit, and again validating David's predicament. Having been heard on this emotional level, David may now be willing to consider the important piece of advice at the end, in vindication of the axiom of "connecting before correcting."

For David to apply for a divorce, on top of losing the ability to walk, in order to avoid the risk of being abandoned and having to accommodate the feelings he expects he would then have, would be an act of experiential *avoidance*. Up until now he has also been *disengaging* by checking out from rehab because he no longer feels able to adhere to his rules for making himself worthy of love. He may not yet be aware that this is what he has been doing, but from the outside, it is fairly easy to see—just as it is to see how a divorce would cause additional stress and magnify the crisis.

In times of crisis, it is judicious to make small decisions and changes. One small but pivotal change happened when David brought his attention and acceptance to his inner experiences instead of putting a lid on them. If he does that once in a while, he will be giving himself the very loving presence he is longing for. He will then have a whole different ball game to play, one that is no longer based in avoidance and self-rejection. Of course, acceptance of "fear of losing love" is not an endpoint. No doubt other emotions will show up: the unfairness of it all, anger, frustration, panic, recurring hopelessness, mourning, shame, and more. A focus on accepting, and even loving, one set of emotions after another, alternating with small, values-based actions designed to address outer circumstances (e.g., rehab), will offer him a way through to acceptance of the whole situation.

In this first meeting with David, acceptance has been introduced as one first important step for him to take. Mindfulness, too, is involved when the psychiatrist and David, together, bear witness to and name the emotions that come up, just as when they named his values of understanding, contributing, and love. In Chapter 2, the psychiatrist mirrored David's "I won't accept being a burden to her" and translated this into positive terms—that is, the value of contributing to his family. She did this because, generally, we are much more likely to come up with solutions and to move in the direction of our values if we have named them in a positive form. Having named the values, the psychiatrist validates David's sinking experiences, such as not knowing how to contribute. Again, she doesn't provide reassurances or solutions at this point but, rather, moves with David to the next level that has opened up: David's misunderstanding that he no longer has anything to offer and the desperate fear he feels when he imagines this circumstance.

We all have misunderstandings about what makes us worthy of love. With awareness, we see them for what they are—misunderstandings. If we sustain the practice of mindfulness and acceptance—with a little coaching if needed—these misunderstandings will, with time, lose their credibility. Therefore, the psychiatrist invites awareness of the misconception and the related fear and pain in order to allow David's tears to flow and his feelings to have all the space they need.

Why should acceptance be one of the main tasks in crisis? Amid the overwhelming experience of something new, unpredictable, challenging, and hazardous, the pull to suppress (and avoid) our inner reactions is very strong—precisely because our inner reactions are so strong. The amplitude of the inner pain scares us. We think we will be swamped if we make direct contact with our feelings. Contrary to what we expect, however, the suppression of inner experience only amplifies our suffering. The paradox is that it is only when we do not try to change our inner response that it *will* change. As we see in more detail in the chapters that follow, it is only through gradually knowing, accepting, and welcoming more of our inner life that our emotional despair will get unstuck and move through us.

Mindfulness

A crisis situation unquestionably needs attention. Mindfulness, the ability to attend to what is going on in the present moment, is the nobility of skills, integral to the two other core processes of acceptance and engagement. Without mindfulness, we are destined to produce our autopilot responses to what's happening, inwardly and outwardly, whereas access to mindfulness can enable us to stay present to events long enough to know and feel our emotions, discover our values, and make conscious, constructive choices (Figure 3–2).

If we can be mindful, even for just a breath, we give ourselves a moment of silence and rest amid the roaring storm of thoughts. Such pauses are often greatly needed. We can wear ourselves down trying to make sense of a situation that doesn't make sense, trying to figure out new ways to get rid of the pain, or entertaining regrets about the past and worries about the future. In this pause and stillness, we can also better recognize and gradually welcome the emotions and bodily sensations triggered by the situation. We foster in mindfulness a state of equanimity that enables us to move between *observing* the pain and *experiencing* the pain and thereby to be less overwhelmed by the pain. Bit by bit, emotional pain can thus be observed, felt, held, and integrated.

By lingering in the present moment, we can learn what matters to us most deeply and evaluate whether the actions we choose are leading us in the direction we want to go. Thus, mindfulness is an integral and es-

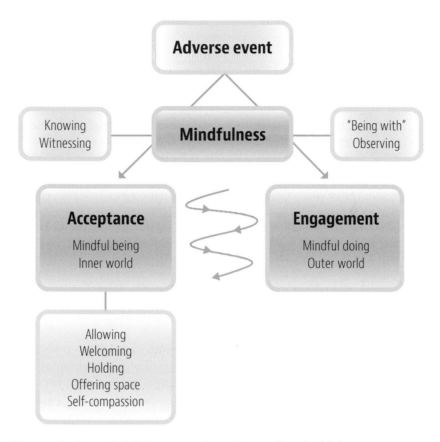

Figure 3–2.   Crisis integration through mindfulness.

sential part of acceptance and engagement: acceptance is "mindful being";
values-based behavior is "mindful doing."

Psychiatrists will be richly rewarded if they cultivate the skill of mindfulness in themselves; it is powerful medicine to be listened to and validated by someone who is 100% present. When the psychiatrist finds it hard
to be mindful, for whatever reason, they can easily follow an impulse to
try to change the patient's distress directly, for example, by correcting or
controlling (e.g., "Try to think this way instead") or by jumping ahead (e.g.,
"It's going to be all right"). Only with full presence, permission, and non-
interference will emotions eventually ease.

To work in the moment, psychiatrists must be able to show up and become aware of what is going on inside themselves before deciding what
action to take, and they must simultaneously be able to attend to the patient and seek to intuit what is happening within them. This is certainly

not easy, and no one we know does it perfectly! But you can aspire to develop the ability to be, and stay, present in the midst of crisis.

Maurice: Clinical Dialogue on Mindfulness

Maurice, a 35-year-old man, had a difficult past involving substance abuse and encounters with law enforcement. When he met the love of his life 2 years ago, however, he straightened up his life and now had a full-time job, was sober, and felt that his life had meaning. Then, one day, he came into the emergency room with a friend. He was upset, with unclear memories of what had lately been going on. His friend told the doctor that both Maurice's girlfriend, Judy, and their baby had died during childbirth 2 weeks earlier. When Maurice was informed about their deaths, he had been offered 3 weeks' worth of benzodiazepines by the gynecologist, but had run out of these before his follow-up psychiatric consultation. He had come to the hospital seeking a prescription for more. In the emergency room, Maurice couldn't recount fully what had happened, and his friend, Johnny, filled in the facts. Maurice may have been suffering the cognitive confusion of an acute crisis reaction (see Chapter 1, "Crisis Fundamentals"), but an inability to consolidate memories can also be an effect of benzodiazepines (Curran 1986; Schatzberg and DeBattista 2019).

It is understandable that a doctor should want to do whatever they can to ease the pain of such a tragedy, but on closer inspection, the use of benzodiazepines may have contributed to emotional avoidance in Maurice. Although one does need respite from the immensity of an event such as this, and sleep is important, as is the need to take things a step at a time, this kind of psychopharmacological intervention introduces the potential for future addiction and risks signaling to the patient that they cannot handle this much pain without medication. Let's see how the dialogue between Maurice and the emergency room psychiatrist develops.

> Psychiatrist: Thank you for filling me in on what happened, Johnny. This is one kind of tragedy that I wish no one *ever* had to undergo. And yet, you are.
> Maurice: I just don't know what to do with myself.
> Psychiatrist: That is *very* understandable.
> Maurice: One minute is like an eternity. I can't stand it! I just need something to knock me out—when I need it, I mean.
> Psychiatrist: I hear you. Time seems endless. What's happened is overwhelming. You want some way of finding rest from it all, at least now and then.

To connect with the patient's reality, the psychiatrist begins by validating Maurice's tremendous loss and his wish for relief.

Maurice: I want more of what the other doctor gave me. Without that, there's no telling what I'll do with myself.

Psychiatrist: I understand from everything you've said that you need some help to be able to get through the day, but I'm also convinced that you will do better without more benzodiazepines.

Maurice: (*in a loud voice*) What do you mean?!

Psychiatrist: I mean that I would be doing you a disservice if I were to pre-scribe benzodiazepines. The problem is that, although benzodiaze-pines will reduce your pain for a while, the pain will come back just as strong afterward. I think you know this. I won't do something that's just going to make you feel worse in the long run.

Maurice: What?! But the other doctor did!

Psychiatrist: I know, I know. The doctor did what doctors sometimes do, which is to use pills when things seem so very difficult. But I know of other approaches that may help you, and I'm sorry, but I'm not going to give you a prescription.

Maurice: (*Stands up, yelling.*) Why not?! What is it that you don't under-stand?

Psychiatrist: (*Silently stays mindful of her own feelings and Maurice's re-action.*)

Maurice: How do you to expect me to get through this without them? I know where to get them, you know, but if I do that, it will get me in trouble. Is that what you want?

Psychiatrist: Certainly not. And I hope you decide not to go in that direc-tion. There are a lot of other ways that I could help you through this terrible, dark time.

In a situation like this, when the patient doesn't receive what they've asked for, there's a risk that they may walk out and that the psychiatrist thus will lose a patient in distress, at least for the time being, but let's see what may evolve should the patient decide to stay.

Maurice: (*Slowly sits down, looks at the floor, and rests his elbows on his knees.*) Yeah, I know they aren't going to fix anything. But the pain— I mean, tell me what else I'm supposed to do.

Psychiatrist: I don't know if I have the one and only answer to this, but one thing you could do, when you feel the wave of pain come over you, is focus your attention on the sensation of your bottom on the chair—that's if you're sitting down—or your feet meeting the ground if you're on your feet.

Maurice: My butt?! (*Looks up at the psychiatrist with disbelief.*)

Psychiatrist: Yes. It's about noticing what you can feel in that part of the body, but in particular where it's in contact with the chair.

Maurice: The one thing I never imagined we'd be talking about right now is how my butt is feeling. But if that's what you want to talk about… (*a tiny smile*)

Psychiatrist: (*with a little smile back*) Sometimes just focusing your attention on one area of your body, such as your bottom or your feet, can give you a more calm and grounded sense of yourself, particularly when such intense emotions are circling around. Would you like to try that?

Maurice: Well, I guess.

As a rule of thumb, for the first month following a severe event, the main emphasis needs to be on stabilization: practical support from others, such as help with everyday chores as well as with new tasks (e.g., organizing a funeral); emotional support, such as hugging and listening or just providing company; and sleeping and eating regularly, taking walks, and keeping up previous helpful routines. While Maurice was grappling with his tremendous loss, it would have been helpful if he'd had access to kindness and care from family and friends around the clock, day and night. However, although he has friends, the reality was that he would probably spend many long hours on his own. The psychiatrist wanted to offer him a self-soothing and calming tool he could use whenever things got really hard. She deployed the "bottom" as possible focus to catch his attention and to evoke a sense of the tangible and down to earth. Sensing that this was not really taking things forward, she directed the focus to his feet.

Psychiatrist: Tell you what, let's forget about the bottom for now. Let's just start with you trying to feel your feet, your feet resting on the floor down there. Will you give that a go? We all know we have feet—I mean, we can see from the outside that we have feet—but that's slightly different from feeling your feet. While you're sitting there, without moving, see if you can sense the shape of your feet, the way they touch the inside of your shoes.

Maurice: What are you talking about?

Psychiatrist: Would you be willing to just try this with me? It may be easier if you close your eyes or—if it feels more comfortable—direct your gaze to your lap for a while.

Maurice: (*Looks down, shaking his head, and after a while closes his eyes.*)

Psychiatrist: Can you feel your feet? How the soles of them feel touching the ground? Maybe you can also feel the toes touching each other.

Maurice: It's even more painful when I close my eyes. Just chaos inside me. Like everything is screaming in panic.

Psychiatrist: It's no wonder, Maurice. And in the midst of that pain, those feelings of chaos and panic, can you feel your feet? Maybe focus on the left one first.

Maurice: The left one…

Psychiatrist: Your left foot—notice how it feels where it meets the sock, the shoe, the floor. (*pause*) Now move your focus to the right foot. Notice where the foot meets the floor. And now see if you can feel that foot, the right foot, from the inside. (*pause*) And then focus

again on any sensations where that foot meets the floor. Feel how
the floor is supporting your right foot. (*pause*) And now do the
same with your left foot.

To have any chance of helping Maurice learn to be with the emotional
thunder of his immense loss, the psychiatrist needs to take things slowly
and enable Maurice to find a calm inner refuge in which he can rest. It is
often useful in mindfulness to begin with the body as the focus of attention, especially those parts at some distance from the torso, which is where
most emotions reside. Resting one's attention on the parts of the body that
are in touch with the floor or the ground may, with time, contribute to a
sense of support. It's a matter of finding out what works best for the individual at that particular moment. The most important thing is to identify
an effective practice that anchors the patient in the present moment and
offers them some tranquility. This anchor can be used to forestall fragmented thinking or to reduce the need to make sense of intense emotional
experiences and somatic responses. An anchor will, with time, improve the
ability to tolerate and connect with what is going on inside.

> Psychiatrist: That's it, feel where your feet are in contact with the floor.
> Then slowly move your attention, nice and slowly, to where your legs
> and bottom meet the chair, the area of interface between you and the
> seat of the chair. Notice how the chair is supporting your weight.
> (*pause*) Now you can move on to notice how your back feels against
> the back of the chair. Allow your attention to settle into where your
> lower back meets the chair. It may help to open that area a little bit
> if we ask Johnny to place his hand on your back. Would that be okay?

Maurice silently nods to give consent to the touch of Johnny's hand,
which may provide an even stronger sense of presence and support than
the chair and thereby help Maurice recognize and accommodate his pain.
The orienting of attention to the areas where Maurice can feel the floor,
the chair, or Johnny's hand is not intended to eliminate, control, or escape
pain. Rather, these points of contact enable grounding, which will give
Maurice a better chance of receiving the pain rather than being consumed
by it and therefore feeling an urge to resist it.

When patients allow themselves to feel the repercussions of a traumatic
event, even for a very short while, they need to know also how to *lean out*
of the pain so it does not overwhelm them. In this example, the psychiatrist
directs Maurice's attention to places outside his torso, both to enable him
to become aware of the present moment experience and to offer him places
where he can lean out of his pain and rest. The practice of acceptance and
mindfulness is not only about feeling and allowing the pain; it's also about

observing it in a non-reactive, tranquil, and compassionate way. To establish such equanimous attention, it's helpful to attend someplace away from the pain—such as the feet, the hands, or sounds—for longer or shorter periods of time. By alternating between *leaning into* the emotional pain and *leaning out* of it, providing space for it, holding it in compassion, we can learn to titrate the immensity of the crisis experience.

In this brief intervention in the emergency room, the psychiatrist aims to strengthen Maurice's holding, self-calming, and resting abilities, as well as his capacity bring awareness to his feelings.

Chapter 5 ("Mindfulness of Body and Feeling") explains in more detail how establishing a mindful perspective will increase our tolerance of emotions and somatic distress during times of extreme difficulty. Chapters 6 ("Acceptance and Self-Compassion") and 7 ("Engagement"), in turn, explore the benefits of cultivating self-compassion and engagement.

Maurice's psychiatrist needs to carefully choose her words and the tone and pace of her voice in order to short-circuit the false sense of urgency that a crisis creates. To bring this kind of calm into her voice, it will be helpful to extend her locus of attention to the same area of her own body while she finds the words to guide Maurice. In a very basic way, the psychiatrist is both modeling and mirroring the mindful processes that are being induced in the patient.

After a little guiding of Maurice's attention to his bodily sensations, he starts to cry, first silently, then more loudly.

Psychiatrist: I can hear the pain in your crying. What is coming up inside right now?

Maurice: I don't know what to do. When is this going to stop?

Psychiatrist: It can be very scary when you don't know what to do, and it feels like this could go on forever. For now, just let yourself feel the pain, the panic, the not wanting it to be this way, the not knowing, just one bit at a time as you become aware of it. See if you can allow whatever comes up to be there. Then notice again the feeling of Johnny's hand resting on your back, kind of supporting you. Just that, just this moment…feeling the pain…and then feeling how your back feels where Johnny has his hand.

Maurice: (*Begins crying and shaking.*)

Psychiatrist: Yes, just let yourself be there with the pain for a little while.

Maurice: (*Stands up and yells at the top of his voice.*) No! No! No!

Psychiatrist: I'm right here with you, Maurice. It's okay to feel what you feel, even if it hurts this much.

Maurice: (*Sits down, crying. Gradually the crying becomes quieter and he becomes calmer.*) What will I do without Judy? How can I live without her? And our little baby? How can I live with this?

Psychiatrist: You're doing it right now.

Maurice: Am I?

Psychiatrist: You can lean in, to feel these intense emotions, to experience the absolute not knowing what to do without these ones you loved so much, and then lean out again—by focusing on your feet on the floor, or your bottom on the chair—to get some rest, and grounding, some space in the turmoil. When you're ready, you can lean into the awfulness of it all once again. One tiny, tiny bit at a time. Just like you are doing.

Maurice: But why would I want to do that? It just hurts so much.

Psychiatrist: What you're doing is a really powerful thing to heal yourself. What I've seen happen, over and over again, is that spending time with the pain creates a different path for you to follow when pain arises. Instead of trying to run away, you have another option at your disposal. When you practice leaning in and leaning out of the pain in the way you just did, your ability to tolerate it will increase, and the pain will become less wild and overwhelming. With time, you will grow inside so that you can offer space for the immensity of it all. You'll no longer be trying to escape it.

Maurice: That seems a long way off for me.

Psychiatrist: And before you reach that point, by all means, take breaks, do whatever will provide you with support, calm, or even distraction, like taking walks in a park or anywhere you can experience nature, or listening to music at home. Please, just avoid drugs, alcohol, or other quick fixes that will only make your pain worse in the long haul. Make sure that you eat and sleep as regularly as you can. Invite a friend to spend some time with you every now and again. I'd suggest you go to work at least part-time to get some structure and company during the day. Also, maybe consider going to a grief support group in the area where you live, or to a community center or church where you might meet some friendly folks. And when that wave of pain comes, don't run from it, just allow yourself a moment to lean in and feel it, then lean out and focus on your feet, say, to steady you.

Maurice: I've never done anything but run away, so I don't know what's going to happen the next time around.

Psychiatrist: Don't expect yourself to be perfect at this. It takes time to practice it and to learn to make room for this amount of pain. Any time it gets too hot to handle, you're welcome to come back here to talk to me or to one of my colleagues. We're open 24/7. We've talked about a lot of new ideas on how to cope with pain, so I'm going to write down a few key ideas and strategies that we've discussed today. Put this on your refrigerator or some other place that you visit regularly during the day, like your bathroom mirror. Okay?

Maurice: Okay. And thank you. I appreciate what you've done with me today.

In this exchange, the psychiatrist supplied a fair amount of structure, even though Maurice was the one doing the work. When thoughts of "I don't know what to do" and "This could go on forever" come up in him, the psychiatrist acknowledged them by reflection, or by naming them, and then guided Maurice back to his body. She coached Maurice to perform certain mindful tasks, such as *being in* and *being with* the inner experiences that appear, practicing a nonjudgmental and non-reactive attitude, and widening his field of attention.

Mindfulness is about more than just creating space to witness inner experiences; it also involves the witnessing of inner bias—that is, observing any aversion to the inner experience or any attachment to what we want the experience to be. These are all basic skills of mindfulness; Maurice is, in effect, now receiving training in mindfulness from the psychiatrist.

In the psychiatric emergency room, security backup will normally be available if a situation should get out of hand. The psychiatrist may nevertheless find it frightening if they allow a patient to express this intensity of pain—"Will I be able to manage this situation?" "Will the patient hurt themself?" They may experience an urgent need to find a way to defuse the situation or may feel perplexed ("What on Earth am I going to do now?") or stressed ("There are a lot more patients in the waiting room"). Indeed, all of these inner reactions can show up at once. As Roberts (2022) noted, difficult experiences with patients "can teach the most important lessons of an entire medical school curriculum but may also elicit feelings of helplessness or distress." At such times, it is essential that psychiatrists be attentive not only to what the patient is experiencing but also to what is going on in themselves. In doing so, they become free to choose how to respond, instead of simply reacting.

As a physician, a psychiatrist is expected to evaluate the patient's state in an ongoing way. If this exercise had been too much for Maurice, she might have chosen to teach him only how to "lean out" of the experience to help to steady him in this acute first phase. In his planned follow-up psychiatric consultation, Maurice would acquire several more tools of self-soothing and be encouraged to recall any strategies he previously practiced, before this catastrophe, to help him soften, feel safe, and calm down. He would also be introduced to techniques such as "diaphragmatic breathing" (Hopper et al. 2019). When he had cultivated equanimity and self-compassion in these and other ways, he would be better able to be with and care for his pain. Because Maurice may develop PTSD or prolonged grief disorder after this loss, those supporting him should be alert at all times for the emergence of new symptoms or unexpected reactions to psychological interventions (American Psychiatric Association 2022; Delaney 2019).

Mindfulness can be integrated into a clinical session in many ways and need not always involve an explicit mindfulness activity of the kind presented here. Mindfulness is in play every time the psychiatrist helps the patient apply a curious and kind attention to what is going on inside them, for example, by reflecting back what the patient says and speculating about the feelings and the unmet needs and values behind the words. In these moments, both the psychiatrist and the patient are attending to several layers of what is happening within the patient. In the acceptance dialogue with David, mindfulness was in play when he was encouraged to remain present long enough to allow his suppressed fear to surface. For Maurice, the psychiatrist modeled acceptance when she encouraged him to stay with his feelings and validated how scary this must be for him. Mindfulness work is, in part, geared toward facilitating acceptance. Mindfulness is similarly a prerequisite to learning about personal values and choosing behavior that serves them. Through such interweaving with acceptance and engagement, mindfulness is central to nurturing flexible responsivity in a changed, painful, and challenging situation.

Engagement

Ultimately, a crisis can't be resolved if feelings are avoided and no actions are taken to solve the problems that need to be solved. *Engagement* is the term from ACT used here to refer to approach-oriented, values-based actions that help patients confront the crisis at hand (Figure 3-3). Engagement always starts with discovering and connecting to our deeply held values. These values center on what we want our life to be about; they are the beliefs and principles we will want to put into motion in a crisis context. In some ways, our values reveal the true source of our inner discomfort. For a life situation to really matter to the patient and to grow to crisis proportions, there must be something important at stake, something for which the patient is seeking or yearning that is not being realized. It may well be that the strategies the patient is using to express their values are actually pushing them further and further away from actualizing them; avoidance behaviors often have this quality. Focusing the crisis conversation on "What are you willing to do differently here that is also consistent with what you want your life to be about?" is a rock-solid intervention strategy. Engagement means formulating strategies that we hope will align with our values and implementing them in the knowledge that doing so may trigger additional emotional pain. It means willingly enacting the chosen behaviors with the intention of accepting any new sources of pain that ensue. Engagement is moreover an iterative process requiring us to gauge the effects of what we have tried and to determine whether these consequences align with our values. If they don't, we then allow these consequences to reshape our behavior. And so it goes on, as larger and larger patterns of engagement are established in our life.

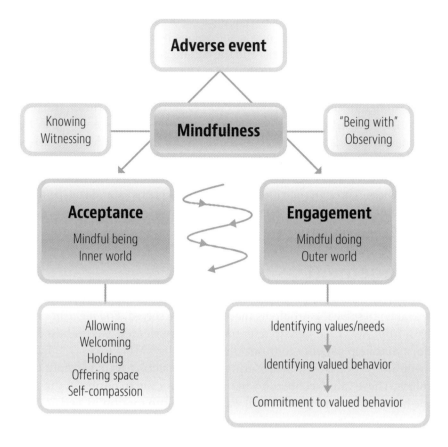

Figure 3–3.   Crisis integration through engagement.

Values are intrinsically motivating and therefore able to regulate be-havior in a wide range of changing life contexts. For example, the value of being honest and forthright could be applied in many interactions. This is why values-based actions are so potent and quick-acting. They can orga-nize wide swaths of patient behavior and are self-reinforcing. At the most fundamental level, values commonly center on love, peace, and wisdom. Other examples of core values are connection, mutuality, integrity, clarity, and purpose. Yet others may vary according to our context: sometimes we value ease and trust, other times inspiration and learning. Values can also be of a very basic kind, for example, caring for our physical being by means of rest and food. Whatever our values, the task is the same: to check in with ourselves, with a sustained curiosity, to discern which of our values are most important for us, both in the moment and in the longer term. When we do this, we are much better able to make good choices about what to do next than when we act according to a set of outdated rules.

It is always a good idea to initiate values-based forms of action, but in the turmoil of a crisis, it is indispensable. When we are fearful or confused, we are particularly prone to rely on rules of behavior that seemed to work well in the past. If these strategies have in some way, however small, contributed to a crisis we now face, then attempting to continue following them will create new problems and add to our confusion. That is exactly what David would find, for example, if he were to apply for divorce because he could see no hope of earning love in the ways he had previously done so. What's needed is to let go of complying with rules and strategies and to shift the focus to underlying needs and values.

When both patient and psychiatrist feel uncertain of what to do next, the clarifying of values will usually get things moving again. Naming values and bringing them into awareness fosters both compassion for the present predicament of not aligning with what is important and guidance for choosing the next step of action. This simplifies what otherwise may look like a complex mixture of different problems to solve and offers a tangible pathway out of crisis. Let us see how this process worked in the second session with David.

David: Clinical Dialogue on Engagement

Psychiatrist: How are you today?
David: I don't know really how to answer that question. But it's good to see you. I've been a bit confused since you last came.
Psychiatrist: Sometimes confusion can be a good thing. Will you tell me more about what's confusing for you?
David: Well, first of all, it's not fun to be me. And having all this time on my own doesn't help. I don't really know what to do with all that is going on in my head.
Psychiatrist: Yes, it's difficult to makes sense of something so big.

The psychiatrist reflects back on and validates David's confusing inner experience. David's tone has shifted from irritability to something more trusting. Without much prompting, he now shares what has been going on for him.

David: I did enjoy seeing my wife and kids yesterday. We had a better time together. Less tension, or something like that.
Psychiatrist: I'm very glad to hear that.
David: And I've been thinking a lot about love.
Psychiatrist: Interesting topic, love, isn't it?

The psychiatrist has made a discreet suggestion that they stay with something that has arisen—by highlighting it as an "interesting topic." It is worthwhile investigating whether a shift in strategies regarding love, a fundamental value, could evolve.

> David: I love them so much. (*He tears up.*)
> Psychiatrist: I know.
> David: I don't want to live without them, but I don't want to be a burden either.
> Psychiatrist: I can hear how difficult those opposing wishes are for you: to be close, on one hand, and to not be a burden, on the other. A very difficult dilemma to navigate your way through.

Again the psychiatrist doesn't contradict David or give answers but introduces a word, "dilemma," to name the aspect of his struggle he has described. It sounds as though David has begun to wrestle with his rules, a step forward that, for now, is exacerbating his sense of confusion. Here the psychiatrist can serve as both a guide and a traveling companion as David explores new terrain, with the intention of giving him space to find his own new answers around the experience of love.

> David: So, what should I do?
> Psychiatrist: I could tell you what *I* think you should do. But that would be rather annoying, wouldn't it? Or at least unsatisfying? What I *can* do, more usefully, is be here for you while you feel your way forward. Someone to bounce ideas off of.
> David: I should have known you'd say something like that.
> Psychiatrist: (*laughing*) Okay, let's get back to where we were—love, yes? Maybe we can look at that from a slightly different angle. As a father, when you think about your children, what would you like them to know—or learn—about love?
> David: I don't know…that I love them?

The psychiatrist helps slow down David's processing of the emotional issues at hand so he can become present to his motives and values. Then she brings the subject of David's children into the conversation. If this gambit—"Think about your children"—is badly timed, the patient may interpret it as a way of inducing guilt, which is rarely helpful. When the timing is right, however, thinking about children can provide a shift in perspective. Seeing his situation through their eyes helps David to step out of his matrix of rules about love. The psychiatrist goes silent to give him time for other thoughts to arise.

> David: Oh, I see what you mean. I can't check out from my family, can I? It wouldn't be a very good example to the kids.

Psychiatrist: Yeah…. In what ways, as you see it, would it not be a good
example?
David: I'm not sure yet, but I realize that it's not an option.

A shift of some sort has happened for David, one that he can't yet put
fully into words. Perhaps he's worked out that checking out from his family would signal that his love for them isn't deep enough to make him stay
with them when the going gets rough. On a slightly deeper level, he may
have meant that if he divorced his wife because he sees himself as unworthy of love now that he is crippled, the message he would be giving his
children would be that love is not unconditional. Or he could mean that,
because of his love for them, he wants to model for his children how to
find a way through times of severe stress. The psychiatrist is now in a position to help him cement one or more of these values-based thoughts.

Psychiatrist: One thing I guess this means is that, because of your love for
them, you want to do what *you* can to stay in the family.
David: (*silence*) I think so.
Psychiatrist: (*silence*) Which would mean that you're willing to risk them
getting annoyed now and then by you being wheelchair-bound, say,
or by your needing help with some basic everyday tasks.
David: I guess so.
Psychiatrist: And that you'd have to get used to the fact that you and your
loved ones would be living in two slightly different worlds—the
world of walkers and the world of wheelchair-users, with all that
that entails.

Hearing this, David sighs deeply and looks down in his lap, with his
shoulders slumped. The psychiatrist spelled out these two painful facts in
order to bring them into David's awareness for present or future acceptance. When David connects to his wish to live a life in love with his wife
and children, he must also be willing to risk exposure to moments when
his family will find his new predicament difficult. He needs to become
willing to open himself to whatever responses may arise (in him or in
them) instead of seeking to avoid such painful situations by checking out
of his marriage and family altogether.

Psychiatrist: But it would also mean that you'll have moments when you
see their eyes light up with love for you, and your heart will light up
with love for them.
David: Do you think so?
Psychiatrist: I do. And this step would mean that you'll be there for them
whenever they need you in the future. You'll be there for them as a
husband and as a dad.
David: (*tearing up*) Yes, I would like that. That would feel good.

The psychiatrist has helped David move toward what he believes in by showing him what can be won by engaging with his difficult circumstances. After this session, David was far more willing to engage with rehab in order to prepare himself for a new kind of life, motivated not by precepts imposed from the outside but by his own authentic aspirations. It had become clear to him why he wanted to come to grips with living his life in a wheelchair. Values may seem lofty and abstract, but in a crisis, it is helpful, when you're choosing what to do next, to remind yourself of what matters the most deep down inside you. When David became unable to adhere to his old strategies, everything seemed pointless; nothing he could do would bring back the capacity to contribute to his wife's and kids' lives in the same way he did before. Yet when he moved from the paradigm of fixed rules—of contributing on a practical and monetary level in order to earn and show love—to the paradigm of love as a value, a door opened to a thousand other possible strategies. Moreover, he was able to find the strength he needed to overcome the many new obstacles he will face in the course of following his values.

When offering guidance to patients in crisis, it helps to have appropriate expectations. You obviously can't change everything in a single session. It's more realistic to see a consultation as propelling a table tennis ball into the situation, a lightweight ball that will bounce around and with time gently shift things, unbinding the patient from unhelpful rules and conditioned responses. It's all the more important to have realistic expectations when dealing with a long-standing crisis, such as we saw Kai undergoing in the previous chapter and whose case we'll return to in Chapter 7, "Engagement."

Alternating Between Acceptance, Mindfulness, and Engagement

No two patients have the same life history or live in the same social and cultural context. Thus, it may seem that no two crises are ever alike. However, the underlying processes that instigate crises are similar, just as the core processes helpful in crises integration are the same. The principles of crisis integration provide guidance through each and every step, boundless learning, and the psychological flexibility necessary to respond to change.

Although it may sound linear when presented theoretically, crisis integration is not a case of one, two, three—mindfulness, acceptance, engagement—job done, crisis resolved. It is more like a spiraling motion that touches in on the three processes again and again, sometimes one at a time, sometimes two at a time, sometimes all three at once. Sometimes people will fall short in this enterprise; other times they will expand their understanding and capabilities.

David's task is to alternate between awareness of the excruciating pain of lost function, together with his fear that his family will lose their affection for him, *and* connecting to his value of love and of contributing to the lives of those dear to him, together with exploring ways to do so. His willingness to face difficult feelings will support him in making choices that are in accord with his values. Vice versa, by connecting with his values, he will find greater motivation to allow his emotional pain and to take the next step, even when his efforts encounter setbacks and disappointments. His mood, sense of agency, self-efficacy, and self-esteem will improve along the way as a result.

Similarly, Maurice's mourning process requires him to find ways to incrementally lean into the depth of his loss while also making room for moments of rest and finding ways to nurture his own well-being. At the same time, he needs to mindfully notice and manage the temptation to escape reality by means of substances, a temptation that may come up a thousand times a day. This will be easier if he can find even the tiniest value to hold on to. What, for example, would his girlfriend have liked to see him doing with his life? How, through his love for her, can he honor her life (and death), moment by moment, day by day?

In our clinical work, we can bear witness to our patients' life crises, even when these are very rocky. We can help them learn how to recognize and hold gently the emotional pain of loss, dismay, torment, or fury that seethes at the heart of a crisis. Even as a crisis is unfolding, we can encourage patients to get past the wish to stifle the distress and pain they feel. The experience of being in torment is not a sign of being broken; it is a sign of being human. ACT helps both psychiatrists and patients take new perspectives on the meaning of personal pain and what to do about it. Instead of seeking ways to reduce the pain, the focus is on increasing one's ability to embrace it.

While attending to present experience and accepting what is going on inside, patients can connect to their needs and advance their ability to behave in ways that provide balance, insight, and health to their lives. They can hold on to deeply held personal values to sustain positive behaviors even in times of emotional pain. Some life events stay with us until the day we die, and the feelings that arise when these memories surface will never be much fun to experience, but they are part of our reality. Committing to make choices based on values both justifies and dignifies the pain. Thus, having a purpose in life helps us accommodate life's unpredictability.

In summary, ACT recasts the definition of the "problem to be solved" in a crisis consultation. It moves the focus away from symptom control or elimination and toward thinking about the patient as a whole person situated in a dynamic life context, in which dealing with crisis is a sort of rite of passage. The goal is to help patients fully know their pain and to serve their highest interests within the changed circumstances that precipitated the crisis. This is what we mean by crisis *integration* as opposed to crisis *intervention*.

References

Acceptance (entry), in Cambridge Dictionary. Cambridge, UK, Cambridge University Press, 2022. Available at: https://dictionary.cambridge.org/dictionary/english/acceptance. Accessed May 16, 2022.

Acceptance (entry), in Macmillan Dictionary. London, Macmillan, 2022. Available at: https://www.macmillandictionary.com/dictionary/british/acceptance. Accessed May 16, 2022.

American Psychiatric Association: Prolonged grief disorder, in Diagnostic and Statistical Manual of Mental Disorders, 5th Edition, Text Revision. Washington, DC, American Psychiatric Association, 2022, pp 322–327

Curran HV: Tranquillising memories: a review of the effects of benzodiazepines on human memory. Biol Psychol 23(2):179–213, 1986 2878691

Delaney S: Grief and loss, in Applied Mindfulness: Approaches in Mental Health for Children and Adolescents. Edited by Carrión VG, Rettger J. Washington, DC, American Psychiatric Association Publishing, 2019, pp 121–134

Hopper SI, Murray SL, Ferrara LR, et al: Effectiveness of diaphragmatic breathing for reducing physiological and psychological stress in adults: a quantitative systematic review. JBI Database Syst Rev Implement Reports 17(9):1855–1876, 2019 31436595

Roberts LW: Learning to care for patients: a comment on "blind spots." Acad Med 97(5):619, 2022 35476827

Schatzberg AF, DeBattista C: Antianxiety agents, in Schatzberg's Manual of Clinical Psychopharmacology, 9th Edition. Washington, DC, American Psychiatric Association Publishing, 2019, pp 421–474

Snyder G: The Real Work: Interviews and Talks, 1964–1979. New York, New Directions Publishing, 1980

Part II

ADVANCED CONCEPTS
AND APPLICATIONS

◇ 4 ◇

A Field Guide to Mindfulness

The education of attention is the education par excellence.

—William James (1890)

Mindfulness: An Inherent Capacity of the Human Brain

Living things were unconscious before some of them became conscious, some 520 million years ago. This evolutionary jump was facilitated by the emergence of a central nervous system with topographical sensory maps of the external world (Feinberg and Mallatt 2016; Frith 2021). Sensory maps provide mental representations of reality so that the conscious subjective experience of an object in the outside world—a tree, for example—is provided by an internal model of that object. This model-based system evolved on top of an earlier model-free system but is by no means unique to humans. The subjective experience of the world is different for, say, a fish, a rabbit, and a human. More complex sense organs—which provide the interface between the neural system and the world—and larger sensory maps process the incoming information in a more detailed way. This adds up to a richer experience of external objects, but the difference is quantitative rather than qualitative (Frith 2021).

Evolution of the human brain also led to a qualitative change, however, in that our brain became able to generate not only subjective experiences of external objects and events and of internal bodily sensations (see Chapter 5, "Mindfulness of Body and Feeling") but also an awareness of having

93

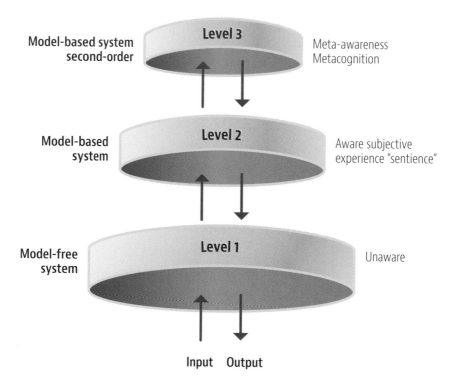

Figure 4–1.   Hierarchy of awareness and of levels of processing.

Source.   Adapted from Frith 2021; Shea and Frith 2019.

these experiences. Humans thus have access to two types of consciousness. The primary type involves an inner representation of the world, what is sometimes called "sentience." The secondary type—or "meta-awareness"—is the awareness of having a subjective experience (Frith 2021; Kabat-Zinn 2019). The experiential implications of the shift of perspective from the first to the second type of consciousness may not at first be obvious but, we hope, will become clear in the course of this chapter and the two chapters that follow.

The human brain also allows us to reflect on experience, as in "thinking about thinking," which is often referred to as "metacognition." We engage in metacognitive activities when, for example, we are determining whether we need to explore further to increase our certainty of what is going on, or to monitor our decision-making procedure (Figure 4–1) (Frith 2021).

These meta-abilities utilize cortical regions developed late in evolution such as the foremost part of the prefrontal cortex, active during planning and decision making; the insula, which supports present-moment awareness of one's own body and emotions; the anterior cingulate cortex, which is involved in directing and regulating attentional focus and in error detection; and the precuneus, a medial part of the parietal lobe that is active during meta-awareness, self-reflection, and other higher-order cognitive functions (Allman et al. 2005, 2010; Bruner et al. 2017; Fleming and Daw 2017; Frith 2021; Kaas 2013; Young et al. 2018). These two meta-abilities—meta-awareness and metacognition—are crucial to finding new and more flexible understanding of and responses to our environment.

It's also on the levels of meta-awareness and metacognition that we find the states and processes of mindfulness. Meta-awareness allows the mindful *observing* of thoughts, feelings, and bodily responses and the knowing of them as such. Metacognitive abilities are applied in the voluntary processes of *directing* attention to present experience, moment by moment. If we look for something more particular than this, we may well miss the simplicity of mindfulness.

Mindfulness is related to the larger field of meditation. *Mindfulness* tends to pertain to a quality of meta-awareness that can be cultivated in everyday life—and advantageously so in clinical settings—as well as in meditational contexts. *Meditation* is a broader concept that includes other practices besides mindfulness for cultivating the mind and is usually practiced formally, as in sitting meditation. Although meditation is at the heart of the mystical traditions of all world religions, mindfulness is not itself mystical. Meta-awareness is available to nearly everyone, at any time; it is an inherent capacity of the human brain. The challenging part is to stay meta-aware of the present moment for longer periods of time. As Sharon Salzberg (2011) put it: "Mindfulness isn't difficult, we just need to remember to do it." In Pali, the language the Buddha spoke, the word *sati* is commonly translated as "mindfulness." It comes from Sanskrit *smṛt*, whose root *smṛ* means "to remember." But how do we remember when we have forgotten? This is where the *practice* of mindfulness comes in. The momentum generated by mindfulness practice will support our ability to stay meta-aware of the present moment for longer stretches of time. With practice, mindful states become more frequent and stable. For some, a crisis may be what it takes to motivate them to learn about mindfulness.

Clinical Relevance of Mindfulness in Crises

Before we further explore what mindfulness is, how it can be practiced, and how it can be applied in clinical work, we need to address an important question: "Why should mindfulness be essential in crisis when there is so much emotional distress and generally so many real-world problems that need to be solved, sometimes urgently?" Mindfulness is sometimes thought of as a luxury for those with the privilege of time and resources. Yet it has been shown that the harsher life is, and the greater the adversities we face, the more beneficial it is to have a practice that brings clarity and rest, expands our capacity to compassionately hold our inner experience, and promotes flexibility in how we respond to hardship (Creswell 2017).

A multitude of randomized controlled trials have provided consistent evidence that mindfulness interventions, relative to treatment-as-usual or no-treatment control groups, reduce depression or relapse rates in individuals at risk, improve substance abuse outcomes, and reduce anxiety and PTSD symptoms. Even those trials that compare mindfulness interventions with gold-standard treatments, such as antidepressant medication, addiction relapse prevention programs, cognitive-behavioral therapy, and prolonged exposure, suggest that mindfulness-based approaches deliver similar or better long-term effects (Creswell 2017). What has also been shown is that mindfulness provides the greatest benefits among high-trauma and high-stress populations (Creswell and Lindsay 2014; Polusny et al. 2015; Williams et al. 2014).

People commonly believe that their internal models based on previous knowledge of the world equate to reality; that their self-instructional thoughts are the truth; that their emotions are either a proper guide for action or harmful states to be suppressed as much as possible. In a crisis, these misunderstandings find leverage. When one relies only on internal reasoning, rules based on prior learning are used to elaborate rules regarding the situation. This manifests as looping thoughts that are seeking a way out yet only become a downward spiral into more suffering and fatigue. When one blindly trusts emotions as a guide for action, what may be seen as trustworthy instinct can, in fact, be biased by prior learning, adding confusion and unnecessary complexity to the situation. Mindfulness, on the other hand, supports accurate perception of the present situation, and this turns out to be far more important than trying to predict the future on the basis of the past.

Mindfulness allows us to perceive thoughts as thoughts, feelings as feelings, and habits as habits, rather than as the whole story. Meta-awareness involves moving out from a state of totally identifying with one's thoughts and feelings. This move, called *cognitive defusion* in ACT, entails a shift of perspective from *within* one's subjective experience to *witnessing* that experience—that is, from the first and second levels of processing to the third level, as pictured in Figure 4–1. This is not to be mistaken for distancing ourselves from experience, or even resigning to it. Rather, it should be understood as an open, allowing, and intentional *knowing* of experience (Yadavaia et al. 2014) that provides a foundation for self-compassion (Neff 2003) and for responding appropriately to situations that do not lend themselves well to verbal-analytic problem solving. The experiences that make up a crisis are the kind that least lend themselves to verbal analysis: invasive, repetitive thoughts; unwanted, distressing emotions; traumatic memories; self-destructive urges; formidable physical sensations. It simply doesn't work to apply socially trained rules and problem-solving methods to such experiences. Attempts to do so will amplify the very things they seek to control.

When what is happening is difficult, chaotic, and painful, as it often is during crisis, it is easy to become immersed in thoughts or emotions, and thus the internal and external reality that currently exists is often only partially known. Most schools of psychiatry and psychology therefore employ *cognitive reappraisal*, by which distorted and unhelpful thinking is identified and then corrected with new, more constructive thinking. This helpfully brings realization that our thoughts do not necessarily present the whole truth. Sometimes, however, cognitive reappraisal exacerbates a mentally arduous situation in which conflicting thoughts struggle to cancel one another out, thereby generating even more thought activity. The simple knowing of mindfulness, on the other hand, involves gentle observation of everything without getting lost in reacting, trying to control, or internally elaborating the content and significance of what's experienced.

The practice of neither fully identifying with inner experiences nor arguing with or judging them is, for many, a new way to relate to experience—one that opens up clarity, acceptance, and freedom in how we respond. The willingness to remain meta-aware of inner events long enough is what enables underlying needs and values to surface. Increased insight into what matters most to us is the foundation of learning to discern which strategies will serve our deepest values and intentions. In this way, mindfulness serves psychological flexibility (Kabat-Zinn 2013).

Various practical tools to promote mindfulness are described in the clinical examples we present in this book, but to become an adept mentor in a clinical context, you need to become well acquainted with mindfulness yourself. This chapter and the next provide a thorough description of mindfulness and exemplify how it can be applied in working with patients. First, however, let us acknowledge a few caveats about any attempt to describe mindfulness.

Experiential Learning of Mindfulness

Most of what we need to know about mindfulness will arise simply from *practicing* mindfulness. When we are mindful, we certainly learn about our present and previous experiences, but we also learn about mindfulness itself—a simple process that paradoxically promises immense and unbounded learning. This is a radically different way to go about learning something. We may be used to studying the world diligently, exercising all our mental faculties to wrap our mind around new conceptual knowledge we want to acquire. When we come to mindfulness and the wisdom it promises, this approach simply doesn't work—a fact that can evoke both frustration and relief.

Ajahn Sumedho, a seminal figure in bringing mindfulness to the West, compared describing the sweet delight of the state of mindfulness to describing the taste of honey:

> That's why you can't do it through thinking or analysis, through defining or acquiring all the knowledge…because although you might know a lot *about* it, you won't know it. It's like knowing all about honey without tasting it—chemical formulas, different qualities, which honey variety is rated the best and the sweetest, which is considered common and vulgar, lower-realm honey. You might know all that but not know the flavour…. But if you just taste the honey, then you are intuitively aware that it tastes like *this*. (Sumedho 2014, pp. 104–105)

Thus, mindfulness is more about experiential than intellectual understanding. This is one of its charms: no authority can teach us fully through words. But we should not underestimate the importance of a teacher or a psychiatrist providing tailored guidance along the way.

Our intention in this book is to offer a description of mindfulness that preempts any impulse to brush it away as mumbo-jumbo or incomprehensible and instead presents it as an accessible and even vital tool in clinical practice. This chapter provides a practical field guide to mindfulness, illustrated with a clinical example of how it can be applied in crisis. Chapter 5 then expands on the mindfulness of body and emotion and its application in crisis integration, again with clinical examples. In this work, we draw on knowledge from cognitive neuroscience and behavioral psychology, intervention research and literature on ACT and mindfulness, and our own clinical experience and mindfulness practice.

Metacognition

It must be made clear that "mindfulness" commonly refers not only to the actual *state* of meta-awareness but also to the metacognitive attentional *processes* of cultivating meta-awareness. The two meanings of the word are not a problem so long as we specify them clearly, as we do in the following discussion, beginning with mindfulness as a process.

Before having a go for ourselves, we might estimate that we could easily stay mindful for at least 10 minutes. Yet when we actually set out to do this, we quickly learn that we forget to remain mindful as soon as after one breath or, at best, five breaths. We start to dwell on things that have already happened, or possibly will happen; our mind unintentionally wanders. This is where the metacognitive mindfulness *processes* come in: the orienting and reorienting of attention upon the present-moment experience; the strengthening of capacity to stay meta-aware of present-moment experience for a longer period. For mindfulness to make a difference, there needs to be some degree of cohesion of attention over time, and any advance in this ability is a major achievement. The practice begins by making use of a set of simple, recognizable metacognitive operations.

Focused Attention

Mindfulness practice commonly starts with developing a focused attention on a single object in the present moment. It doesn't matter to which object we choose to attend; what we are after is simply the cultivation of steady attention over time. At the outset, however, it's wise to choose something that is relatively easy to stay with without getting lost in intense emotions or elaborate thinking. One common such object of mindfulness is the breath. Although mindfulness is not to be mistaken for a breathing exercise, the breath offers movements in the torso on which attentional processes may be anchored.

The breath is not everybody's ideal first choice, however; for one patient, listening to her own breath reminded her of hearing her grandfather's breath when he was sexually abusing her. When breath has come to signify a terrible experience, another focus of attention is obviously preferable, such as sounds in the physical surroundings, tastes of food, sensations in the feet when walking slowly, or anything else that is happening in the present moment.

Whatever focus is chosen, the mindfulness process applies to the same manifold cognitive operations of *selecting, orienting*, and *directing* attention to the focus object; *sustaining* attention on the object for a prolonged period, even in the presence of distractions; *monitoring* when attention floats away in wandering thoughts or other distractions; *comparing* the nature of present mental activity with that of the mindfulness instructions; *detecting* any clinging to distractions; *moving* attention away from distractions; *noting* any reactivity or internal criticism with respect to having been distracted and introducing an *accepting* stance; gently *shifting* and *directing* attention back to the object of focus, again *sustaining* attention on the object, and so repeating the process.

Whether we perform these cognitive operations in our own mindfulness practice or by way of guiding our patients, the intentional choosing of where to direct attention makes use of so-called top-down processes.

Bottom-Up and Top-Down Modulation of Attention

When the outer world bombards us with stimuli—sights, sounds, touches, tastes, smells—and the inner world is swirling with activity—thoughts, emotions, bodily sensations—it is easier said than done to choose what we attend to. To learn more about the ways attention can be directed, let us return to Figure 4–1.

Stimuli that are especially effective in grabbing our attention are those that have gained emotional salience through previous learning. We are all acquainted with the power that nice things and nasty ones—good food, an appreciative smile, or angry eyebrows—as well as new and unexpected stimuli can have on our attention. As mentioned in Chapter 2, "The ACT Model of Crisis Instigation," our brains are wired to gear our attention toward what has been important for our species' survival (through evolutionary learning) or for our personal thriving (through model-free and model-based learning). When attention is caught—and neural information-processing is elicited—by incoming sensory stimulation that is in concert with previous learning, attention is said to be directed via "bottom-up" processes. The information is processed on Levels 1 and 2 in Figure 4–1. This is what advertisers exploit in any way available: blinking, colorful, primordial images with a magnetic pull on our attention. Attention is an extremely valuable currency—which should be as good a motivator as anything for us to learn more about it.

Even when we close our eyes to engage with our inner world, previously encountered events and our models about them will circulate in almost perpetual motion. Luckily, we have the option to choose which things we attend to and which we ignore by accessing a top-down direction of attention, as in the selecting, orienting, and sustaining described earlier (Frith and Dolan 1997).

Tasks such as solving a mathematical problem or sailing in a shallow bay also engage Level 3 in Figure 4–1 and direct attention to *goal-oriented* information-processing and action. In other words, attention is directed to that which is relevant to a predetermined objective. In mindfulness, however, we have *no goal* other than to know what is going on in the present, moment by moment. Yet the manifold top-down attentional operations we use are similar in both instances.

Open Attention

Once we have repeatedly reoriented our attention to the present moment, there will come a time when mindfulness happens effortlessly for longer sweeps of time. Mindfulness, like anything we practice, becomes easier over time.

As the continuity of meta-awareness of present-moment experience stabilizes and strengthens, we may maintain a focused attention on our chosen object of mindfulness, such as the breath, in order to rest in a calm, unreactive state. In crisis, it is particularly beneficial to nurture this kind of soothing state of meta-awareness and to know that it is always available.

We also have the alternative of ceasing to attend to such a "primary" object of mindfulness and opening our attention to observe any experience that happens to show up. In principle, our attention is then free from reference, choice, and fixation and is open to receive and include anything that arises. We aim not to dwell on the experiences that happen; they are allowed to come and go without any attempt to hold onto or suppress them, to grasp or avoid. If at any point we should get lost in our thoughts, we may again use our top-down cognitive processes and bring our attention back to our primary object of mindfulness for a while. After reestablishing in this way a meta-aware outlook, we are better able to remain meta-aware of thoughts *as* thoughts rather than getting absorbed in their content. The same is true for feelings; we can observe them instead of being overwhelmed by them.

Meta-Awareness

Just as the skills of mindfulness are learned and strengthened gradually, so does the knowing of the mindfulness state unfold over time. Even those who dedicate their lives to meditation and teaching mindfulness will refine their description of mindfulness as the decades pass by. This is hardly mystifying, because mindfulness "emerges through paying attention on purpose, in the present moment, non-judgmentally to the unfolding of experience moment-by-moment" (Kabat-Zinn 2003, p. 145). The key word here is *through*. *Through* reestablishing attention in the way described, the mindfulness state arises. Practice of mindfulness brings about continuous discovery of new richness and nuance. Thus, the many definitions of mindfulness reflect the different learning, training, and stage of development of those who offer them. They may also be shaped according to the level of experience of those to whom instruction is being directed.

Nevertheless, there are *three* dimensions that definitions of the mindfulness state often boil down to—each necessary, and together sufficient (American Psychiatric Association 2022; Goldstein 2013; Yadavaia et al. 2014): 1) experiencing what is in the present moment; 2) meta-awareness of the present-moment experience; and 3) meta-awareness of any filter through which the present moment is observed (Figure 4–2). Let's expand on these qualities one by one.

What's the Present Moment Got to Do With It?

Our pets are good at reminding us what being in the present moment is about (Goldstein 2020). A dog follows its nose and responds promptly to ever-changing scents that appear on a walk. It doesn't seem to dwell on the past or worry about the future; instead, it eagerly follows each moment's alluring odor. When we come home to our canine friend, he wags his tail and rejoices rather than residing in resentment because he's been left alone. This capacity to fully experience the present moment is an attractive quality that we can both love and envy. Why would we not want some of a dog's simplicity of response to the world, as it is right now, moment to moment?

However, although our dog's attention is in the present moment, it is not particularly mindful (Goldstein 2020). The processes responsible for his experience and choices happen on the first and second levels of processing in Figure 4–1. Incoming sensory stimuli capture the dog's attention based on his evolutionarily wired nervous system and its previous knowledge. His attention is directed via bottom-up processes—that is, it is mainly stimulus driven.

Meta-Awareness of Present-Moment Experience

The next necessary quality of mindfulness is meta-awareness of the present moment: the *knowing* that we are having an experience; a movement from only *feeling* despair, for example, to also *observing* despair. This refers to the two levels of consciousness introduced at the beginning of this chapter and illustrated in Figure 4–1: the subjective experience (Level 2) and meta-awareness of the experience (Level 3).

This shift of perspective to meta-awareness involves a form of defusion, disembedding, coming loose from experience, that sometimes takes a bit of resolve—especially when it comes to thinking. It often seems as

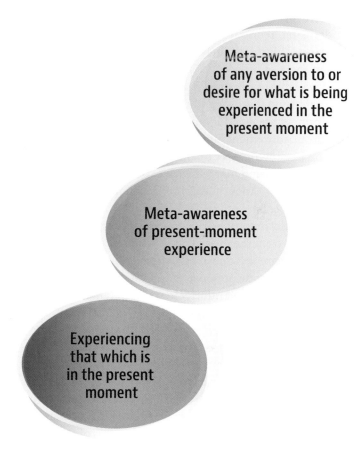

Figure 4–2.   Three dimensions of mindfulness.

though we're glued to thinking thoughts: "I will just think this one train of thought first" or "I really need to figure this thing out first." We're so accustomed to thinking that we sometimes unwittingly presume that even mindfulness means thinking. But mindfulness is different from thinking about thinking—contemplating, reflecting, evaluating, conceptualizing, categorizing, and associating *about* what is being experienced. In other words, mindfulness is different from being immersed in thoughts about the present-moment experience. Mindfulness, in the sense of meta-awareness of thoughts, means recognizing thoughts merely as "thoughts."

The role of metacognition needs to be clarified here. Yes, metacognition does also encompass thinking about thinking, which is sometimes very helpful. However, metacognition applied to the process of mindfulness concerns merely the orienting of attention to the present moment, recognizing when this is not happening, remembering the mindfulness instructions, defusing, reorienting attention to the present-moment experience, and so on. This mindfulness process is what eventually supports longer periods of meta-awareness.

Defusion is available at any time, in any place, but it is crucial to know that, usually, we must do this over and over again. We may mistakenly believe that mindfulness has failed if our attention wanders off, but there is no once-and-for-all movement into meta-awareness of experience for anyone. Defusion is something we do on repeat, and it requires much patience. We defuse from being merged with experience and move into observing it. Then, before we know it, this merging happens again—until we notice that it has happened.

To overcome the stickiness of being immersed in experience, we cannot abandon or turn away from the experience—whether thoughts, emotions, or sensations. Meta-awareness doesn't equate to being a disengaged spectator. It is, rather, a soft, gentle presence to experience. Think of your interested and alert observation of a butterfly in your open hand. As we explore in greater depth in Chapter 6, "Acceptance and Self-Compassion," meta-awareness is one of the foundations of self-compassion. The movement from being merged with experience toward meta-awareness of it is sometimes referred to as "letting go." Jack Kornfield (2008) wrote, "To let go does not mean to get rid of. To let go means to let be. When we let be with compassion, things come and go on their own." When the butterfly is ready, it can take off from our open hand and from our gentle meta-awareness.

As we explore in depth in Chapter 6, meta-awareness of experience also entails noticing and eventually unhooking from any identification with the experience. To give a simple example: "I am afraid" is noticed as fear and identification with fear; it is eventually reframed as "fear is happening" or just "fear." In ACT language, this involves a shift from being defined by the *content* of experiences—called "self-as-content" ("*I am* afraid")—to being the *observer* of the content, or "self-as-context" ("there *is* fear"). Self-as-context means having a sense of self as the perspective from which life is experienced, to be distinguished from one's identity (Yadavia et al. 2014). This will ease strong personal attachments to beliefs, thoughts, and emotions. Non-identification thus also decreases reactivity—the impulse to interfere with and change experience—while increasing the capacity to receive the present experience, as it is, with equanimity and compassion. Ajahn Chah (1918–1992), a Thai forest monk, gave this simple meditation instruction: "Become the witness of it all, the person with perspective, the One Who Knows" (Kornfield 2021).

Meta-Awareness of Any Aversion to or Desire for What Is Being Experienced in the Present Moment

The third quality necessary for mindfulness is to be meta-aware of any filter through which we attend to our experience. Are we observing our experience with an ever-so-slight aversion—wanting to avoid it, judge it, push it away, get rid of it? Or, contrarily, is there any desiring to have more of it, move toward it, grasp it? These pulls in opposite directions correspond to the avoidance–approach system of any organism, all the way down to single-celled creatures. As discussed in Chapter 2, this system has evolved as a means of guidance to sustain life in relating to outer events. However, unaware grasping for pleasant inner experience (e.g., happiness) and blind rejection of unpleasant inner experiences (e.g., anxiety) will both get us into trouble. Avoidance of inner events is what most commonly must be dealt with among those in crisis, but as we will see in Chapter 5, clinging to happy inner states is also problematic.

The Buddha didn't teach a belief system to which one must ascribe; rather, he described his understanding of how the mind works and encouraged his listeners to confirm its validity for themselves. He regarded the unaware tendencies to approach or avoid experiences as a basis of suffering. He suggested that personally exploring the push and pull of aversion and grasping can deliver freedom from these deeply conditioned tendencies and, further down the line, facilitate wise discernment and a path toward peace.

Nurturing non-reactivity and non-attachment in mindfulness does not mean trying to get rid of the aversion or desire. That would be just another level of rejection—now of the aversion or desire. Instead, it means noticing and knowing the inner tendencies of push and pull. The same principle of observing and non-interference is thus applied also to the inner phenomena of bias and preference. Mindfulness is, in the end, not about rejecting; it is about recognizing—seeing things for what they are.

Rather than controlling these inclinations or acting upon them, this *knowing* of wanting less or more plays a major role in reducing affective reactivity. What we come to learn is that meta-awareness of our habitual approach-and-avoid system will, with time, generate an attitude of equanimity toward the content and charge of experience. When we are meta-aware—not only of our present-moment experience but also of what we want *to do with* our experience, avoid it or approach it—we begin to close in on the ambrosia of mindfulness.

The shift from acting on to merely observing these tendencies fosters calm, which in turn makes it easier to discern more aspects of what is arising in the present moment. Mindfulness becomes thereby an *iterative* process through which we become increasingly meta-aware of our subtle, and not so subtle, tendencies to avoid and cling to inner experiences. In other words, we become, with time, more able to notice when meta-awareness of an experience is blended with an ever-so-slight wish for this present experience to stay or go away. Our skills in inner observation will help to neutralize our efforts to struggle against or change experiences so that we can save that energy for more productive endeavors. In Jon Kabat-Zinn's (2016) words: "Meditation is the only intentional, systematic human activity which at the bottom is about not trying to improve yourself or get anywhere else, but simply to realize where you already are." The paradox is that mindfulness or meditation can in the end build the very capacities needed to change those outer circumstances that *can* be changed.

With these three necessary and, together, sufficient aspects of mindfulness (Goldstein 2020)—being in the present moment, meta-awareness of the present moment, and meta-awareness of any desire to change the present inner experience—we can gain a clear understanding of the complete picture of reality as it is offered in the moment.

As our mindfulness practice evolves, we will be able to fluidly move back and forth between sustaining meta-awareness with and without a specific focus. A watermark moment is when we find that, whatever the experience may be, our meta-awareness of it remains unaltered (Goldstein 2013). We can hold in meta-awareness experiences that are painful, neutral, or joyful—whatever presents itself—without losing that meta-awareness. With more frequent moments of leaning into and residing in meta-awareness, we will eventually find it to be a precious restful place amid the turbulence and chaos of a crisis. A calm, allowing, alert meta-awareness.

Abiding in meta-awareness is a listening of sorts. When we listen to birds sing, we cannot make the birds sing in a certain way; we are just witnessing, carefully listening.

Someone once asked Mother Teresa what she said to God when she prayed. "I don't say anything," she replied. "I just listen." The interviewer then asked what God said to her, to which she responded, "He doesn't say anything. He just listens." With her characteristic candor, she added, "And if you don't understand that, I can't explain it to you" (Goldstein 2013). Psychiatrists don't get off the hook that easily. Therefore, in the discussion that follows are some practical examples of how mindfulness can be explored in crisis (see also Figure 4–3).

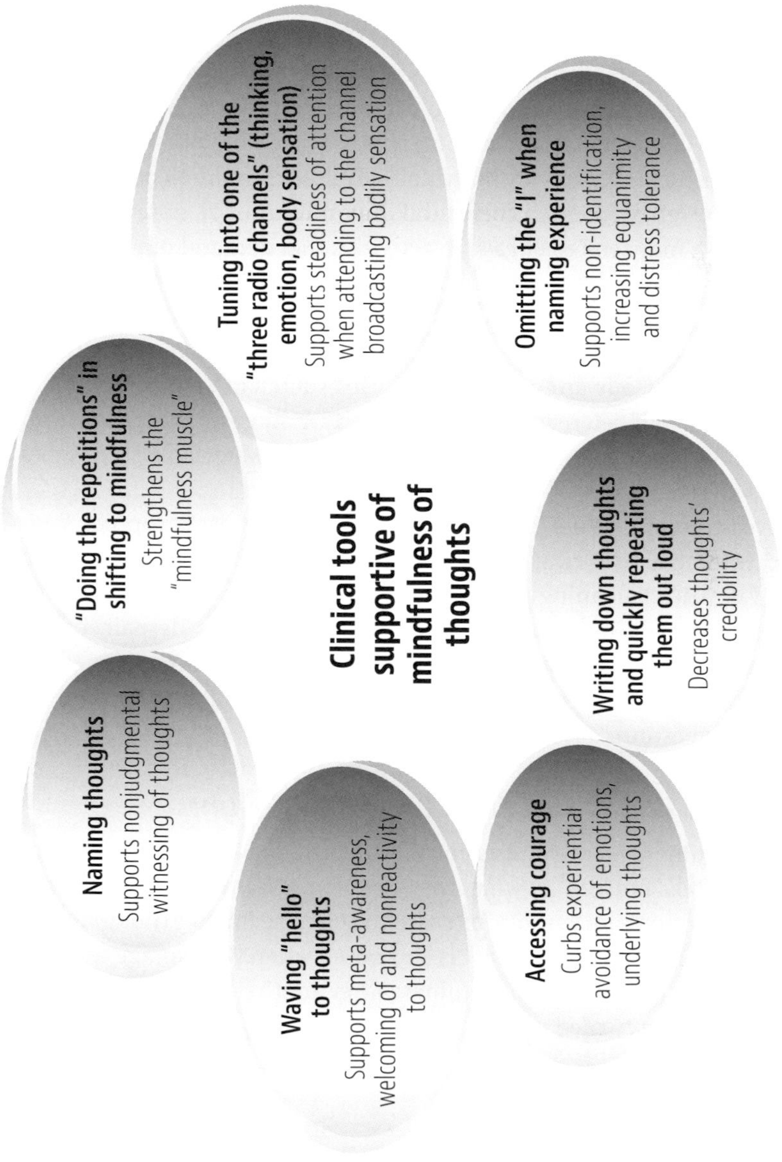

Tuning into one of the "three radio channels" (thinking, emotion, body sensation)
Supports steadiness of attention when attending to the channel broadcasting bodily sensation

Omitting the "I" when naming experience
Supports non-identification, increasing equanimity and distress tolerance

"Doing the repetitions" in shifting to mindfulness
Strengthens the "mindfulness muscle"

Clinical tools supportive of mindfulness of thoughts

Writing down thoughts and quickly repeating them out loud
Decreases thoughts' credibility

Naming thoughts
Supports nonjudgmental witnessing of thoughts

Waving "hello" to thoughts
Supports meta-awareness, welcoming of and nonreactivity to thoughts

Accessing courage
Curbs experiential avoidance of emotions, underlying thoughts

Figure 4–3. Clinical tools to support mindfulness of thoughts.

Crisis Integration Through Mindfulness of Thoughts

We invest a lot in our thoughts. We believe them and identify with them. We try to figure out solutions to the problems they present. In times of distress, we ruminate on the past, worry about the future, or blame and judge ourselves or others. Yet the many means of distraction by which people try to sidestep thought activity, such as entertainment, screens, or substances, would appear to suggest that thinking is not a desirable pursuit. Participants in one study even preferred to self-administer mild electric shocks rather than be left alone with their thinking (Wilson et al. 2014). Distractions aside, we may seek to engage in activities that demand our total cognitive capacity. Many describe difficult or even dangerous pursuits such as playing chess, climbing, performing surgery, or making high-voltage electrical repairs as providing a welcome pause in ordinary thought activity. The absorption of our attention in activities such as these brings relief from our usual self-referential mental activity, a kind of "vacation from ourselves." When it is over, however, the familiar waterfall of thoughts picks up where it left off.

In crisis, emotions are intense and thoughts are catastrophic, fragmented, intrusive, looping, and exhausting. Thoughts such as "Everything is lost," "Life has no meaning anymore," "I cannot stand this," "It is my fault," or even "I deserve this" produce painful emotions—fear, despair, panic, guilt, shame—that stimulate further thoughts along the same lines. Buddhists call this phenomenon *papañca* (in Pali), which roughly translates as "mental proliferation."

Mindfulness Brings Rest From Looping Thoughts

When mindfulness is introduced into this whirlpool, thoughts and emotions are merely noticed as what they are. For a moment, the agitated thoughts and importune emotions cease to generate further thoughts and emotions. A sense of ease and rest is cultivated when we manage to experience one such moment of mindfulness after another. This is something to be glad about. It turned out to be a helpful first step for a patient called Marina.

Marina: Clinical Dialogue on Resting From Looping Thoughts

Marina is a 30-year-old single woman and a second-generation immigrant. She learned through partner tracking at age 23 that she had HIV. She didn't complete her college education, and at present she has no job. Her waking hours are tormented by thoughts about being HIV-seropositive that erode her ability to focus on anything else. In addition to a continuous sense of shame and self-loathing, she struggles with a prevailing sense of loneliness and meaninglessness. Today's antiretroviral medications are excellent, yet Marina, like others, suffers because of the stigma of her condition. She fears she would lose a large part of her social network if her HIV diagnosis were known. Many people living with HIV dare not tell anyone, or tell only a very few trusted individuals. The risk of becoming a social outcast if the truth were revealed is perceived as unbearable, but the secrecy, too, creates a sense of loneliness, a sense of living a double life.

This risk of social rejection has become for Marina an ongoing crisis. When the only friend of hers who knew about her disease committed suicide a few months ago, the pressure of her own suicidal thoughts increased. If her friend, who didn't even have HIV, decided to kill himself, then why should she want to live?

The psychiatrist is meeting with Marina for the first time after her HIV health care contact referred her on account of her depression and suicidal ideation.

Psychiatrist: So what would you say is most difficult for you in all of this?
Marina: It's hard to say. I feel haunted by HIV all the time. It's the first thing I think of when I wake up and the last thing before I fall asleep. Even during the night I wake up thinking about it.
Psychiatrist: It must be exhausting.
Marina: I'm so tired.... Well, it's weird—I feel kind of really tense, but also totally drained, as if I couldn't move a limb. And the thoughts, they don't let up, even for a moment. I just don't know what to do with myself.
Psychiatrist: Can you tell me what these thoughts are like, what they're about?
Marina: Okay. You know, HIV (*sighs*) Where do I start? Nobody likes someone with HIV. If my friends knew, they'd all dump me. They tell me I'm beautiful, that they love me. But they don't know. My life is one—big—lie. (*quietly*) I just feel so lonely. I sometimes go to parties, but people wonder why I always turn guys down. Even nice ones. I don't know what to say anymore. It's kind of easier to stay home, but at home I'm alone with my thoughts again. The TV is the only company.
Psychiatrist: So, if you were to tell the truth of your diagnosis, you'd become alone for real, and if you don't tell the truth you're alone in a different way.
Marina: Exactly. Although I've been debating whether I should tell the truth and see what happens. If it turned out to be as bad as I fear, I could move to a different town and start over. But, then again, it would only be a matter of time before my HIV would catch up with my new life. I know I would be fearing that scenario all the time.
Psychiatrist: It's a difficult situation indeed. And your thoughts, they're working hard to try to find a way out, am I right?
Marina: For years. Day after day. They never stop.

> Psychiatrist: And who can blame them? Your thoughts, I mean. We are social animals. To lose the social support of our clan is one of the most dangerous things that can happen. We're programmed to feel really scared of such social rejection.
>
> Marina: (*Looks down at her hands and begins to shake and sob. Tears begin running down her cheeks.*) Yes,...I'm scared.

In suspecting and suggesting that the situation threatens the universal need to be included and safe, to belong, the psychiatrist has sought to help Marina understand that it makes perfect sense to feel scared, and how this fear will trigger thought and problem-solving activity. Giving voice to needs and emotions promotes a meta-awareness of them, and the hope is that it will spur Marina's acceptance of her looping thoughts as she tries to figure out what she should do. Now that this level of needs, feelings, and thoughts has been named, the next level of thoughts—ones of self-accusation and concomitant feelings of shame and guilt—can surface into awareness.

> Marina: Having HIV means you're disreputable, cheap—sullied.
>
> Psychiatrist: Is that what your thoughts are telling you?
>
> Marina: Well, no, that's what I *am*. It's my fault! If I hadn't had unprotected sex with this guy, I wouldn't be here. It's like I'm a slut.
>
> Psychiatrist: So the story by which you try to make sense of this painful situation is that it's your fault because you are a slut. Is that how it works?
>
> Marina: (*with some hesitation*) Yes...I guess that's it?
>
> Psychiatrist: To put this in perspective, you're not the only person in history who's had unprotected sex. Probably most people have done the same thing at some time in their life. You were just unlucky.
>
> Marina: (*Takes a long look into the psychiatrist's eyes.*) But...

In this interchange, the psychiatrist has set the stage for a more objective and self-compassionate way in which Marina could relate to herself. Marina's resistance to that is evident in her "But...." The psychiatrist interrupts her:

> Psychiatrist: I doubt I'll have any luck persuading your thoughts to take a rest if I try to reason with them. The thoughts also won't change their opinions that easily, will they?
>
> Marina: No.
>
> Psychiatrist: I just wanted you to consider that there may be any number of stories about what's happened to you that would seem to make sense and be logical. What I think we need to do now is to help you relate to your thoughts in such a way that they don't consume all of your energy. I'd like you to be

able to access a bit more stillness of mind and, indeed, a bit more rest in general. Would you be interested in hearing what I have in mind?

Here the psychiatrist puts words—*rest* and *stillness*—to values Marina has implicitly brought up when describing how her incessant thoughts wear her down. Putting values on the table could possibly increase the motivation to try something new. Marina agrees to hear what the psychiatrist has to suggest.

> Psychiatrist: One way of neither agreeing nor disagreeing—neither getting involved and expanding on the thoughts nor battling with them—would be just to notice that these thoughts are occurring.
> Marina: What?
> Psychiatrist: I mean noticing that "thoughts are happening; thinking is like this." I'm guessing by the look on your face that what I'm saying doesn't make much sense. Shall we just try it? That's probably easier than trying to explain it.
> Marina: I have no idea where you're going, but okay.

Thoughts typically don't respond well to efforts to change them, irrespective of whether they are true or false, or right or wrong. The very act of trying to change, control, or eliminate thoughts tends to make them proliferate, so they become even more intrusive. Such efforts are likely to have played a major role in escalating Marina's depression and suicidality. Moreover, she might well actually experience what she fears most—being rejected by her friends and regarded as sullied—if she were to reveal her predicament. She can, however, turn inward in search of acceptance, compassion, and rest.

One step in this direction is being able to notice one's thoughts as thoughts. Accessing meta-awareness in this way supports the ability to receive and accept what is going on within. To shift from being completely merged with her thoughts (Level 2 in Figure 4-1) to simply observing them (Level 3), Marina needs to detach from their content, even if only a little. Since thoughts are by nature captivating and incredibly enticing to pursue or to argue with, this is not easy.

In an analogy of Goldstein's (2013), thoughts, emotions, and body sensations are broadcast on three different radio channels: channel 3 broadcasts thinking; channel 2 broadcasts emotions; and channel 1 broadcasts body sensations. Channel 3 is the most challenging one to remain mindful toward because it's so easy to be swept away by thoughts. It's easier to remain mindful about what's happening on channel 2 and even easier to sustain steady attention on the body sensations of channel 1. In crises, when busy inner activity is the rule rather than the exception, it is helpful to tune into channel 1 rather than channel 2 or 3. For this reason, the psychiatrist chooses the movement of breath as Marina's first mindfulness object. Meta-awareness of the breath will eventually support her ability to be meta-aware of thoughts when they show up, instead of believing in and elaborating their content.

> Psychiatrist: Thank you. Now, this kind of thing is sometimes easier when you're not distracted by vision. If you feel comfortable doing so, I suggest you close your eyes. Or else just keep your gaze soft and directed to your lap. Now, check if you can sense your breath. Take a deep breath in, if you will, and notice how your belly feels as you breathe in. Does the belly expand forward, sideways, even backward on your in-breath? Does it relax on your out-breath? (*pauses*) If it's easier, you can choose to feel the breath in your chest. Notice how your ribs expand and separate on your in-breath (*inhales*), and settle back in place on the out-breath (*exhales*). In-breath…and out-breath…. How are you doing?
>
> Marina: Okay. I'm breathing.
>
> Psychiatrist: Great. Keep noticing your breath. As best you can, follow the in-breath, how the breath peaks and turns, and the out-breath…. Even with the best of intentions to stay with your breath, a thought will probably sooner or later sneak in. That's close to being a law of nature. When that happens, will you let me know?
>
> Marina: Well, for a start, I'm wondering where all this is leading.
>
> Psychiatrist: Splendid. So now you can try this: instead of internally answering this question—whether it's "This is leading nowhere" or "Give this guy a chance"—would you try just waving hello to the thought? Wave hello to the thought of "Where is all this leading?"
>
> Marina: You mean I should actually wave?
>
> Psychiatrist: If that helps, or you can just imagine waving. Wave hello to the thought "Where is all this leading?" Can you do that?
>
> Marina: I don't know. It sounds a bit strange to me.
>
> Psychiatrist: Okay, that's fine. Let's try another way of responding to the thought.

The psychiatrist provides Marina with a couple of tools for staying in mindfulness when channel 3 comes on again after she has tuned into channel 1. One is to invite and welcome the thought by waving at it. Another is to give the thoughts each a nickname. Explicitly welcoming a thought orients your attention to what is being welcomed. "Naming" supports a nonjudgmental witnessing of any subjective experience that appears. The experience need not be thoughts; the method can be applied also to emotions or bodily sensations. Examples of naming some experiences during this practice could be: "catastrophic thoughts," "fear," "heart beating." These techniques counteract two common tendencies of getting lost in, expanding on, or overidentifying with inner experiences *or* of avoiding them. They support a shift to being meta-aware of them.

> Psychiatrist: How about just giving the thought "Where is all this leading?" a simple name like "thought" or "thinking is like *this*"? Or you could name the related feeling—say, "meaninglessness." And after you've named the thought, or feeling, you go back to the breath.
>
> Marina: Okay.
>
> Psychiatrist: Wonderful. Sensing how the belly or the chest gradually expands on the in-breath (*inhales*) and relaxes on the out-breath (*exhales*). Feeling the sensations of the beginning, the middle, and the end of the breath as well as the space in-between the breaths. Bringing a caring attention to this wave of sensations.
>
> Marina: I'm feeling so tired, so weary.
>
> Psychiatrist: I understand. Tired, weary…. Would you be happy to name aloud the tiredness, the weariness? Just to have a go at that?
>
> Marina: Okay…. Tiredness. Weariness.
>
> Psychiatrist: Beautiful. And as you name these experiences—acknowledge them—you can even gently welcome them. And then you return to the breath, feeling how the belly—or the chest, whichever is easier—moves with each breath.
>
> Marina: If I have the thought that my HIV means I'm sullied, do I have to welcome that as well? That sounds…I don't know… like it'll just make it worse.
>
> Psychiatrist: It's good that you bring this up. What I would suggest is that as soon as you notice there's an "I" in a thought, you drop the "I." So "I am sullied" will become "thought about sullied" or "self-judging thought." Or you could name the feeling caused by the thought—maybe "shame," for example. Or simply "painful thought" would do. To give another example: "I am scared" could translate as simply "fear." How does that sound? Would that make it simpler to welcome these thoughts?
>
> Marina: I don't know. It sounds awkward.
>
> Psychiatrist: When you say "awkward" I wonder if what you mean is that it's something you're unaccustomed to. Would that be true? If we can step beyond that, I would be curious to know whether you might feel less need to struggle with the content of your thoughts if you were to realize that what you're thinking doesn't actually define who you are. And less struggle means more rest.

To facilitate letting go into meta-awareness and to reduce the stickiness and pull of experiences, it is useful to name the internal processes without using the pronoun "I." When experiences are no longer attached to a "me," they become less threatening because they neither describe a "me" as a person nor belong to a "me." This enables *reactivity* to decrease in the midst of crisis and *tolerance of distress* to increase. Mindfulness involves moving from the narrow perspective of identifying with thoughts to a wider perspective of observing. We move beyond what previous learning has defined us to be and lean into knowing, receiving, and embracing the pain of a crisis. We are the pain, but we're also something bigger than the pain.

> Psychiatrist: So, again, feel your breath—notice how the sensations of the breath arise, change, and dissolve. And, if you're willing, please name anything that comes up.
> Marina: I'm thinking about being sullied again—or, I guess, a thought about being sullied has come up.
> Psychiatrist: A thought of being sullied arises. Thank you. Now bring your tender attention back to the movements of your breath. Noticing the beginning, middle, and end of each breath.
> Marina: (*after a little while*) I just feel so bad, so ashamed, like I'm sinking.

Although Marina has beautifully omitted the "I" when referring to the sense of being sullied, she is still partly identifying with this concept. One cannot expect complete disidentification to happen in one go. Nevertheless, Marina is now able to move on to the feelings that the thoughts about being sullied have inspired. These feelings may actually be what she first encounters when she momentarily lets go of thinking about being sullied.

> Psychiatrist: A feeling of being ashamed showed up, as if you were sinking. See if you can stay with that for a while and give some company to this shame and sinking.
> Marina: Okay. (*pause*) I just don't know what to do. There's nothing I can do.
> Psychiatrist: The despair of not knowing what to do, not knowing anything that will help.... Now see if you can gently go back and offer the shame a little company. Nothing to do now, nothing to become, just offer company to the shame. And, if you can, bring a curious, friendly attitude to the shame and the sinking.

When you encounter a highly uncomfortable feeling, such as shame, it is common to want to *do* something, to find a lever that could catapult you out of the feeling. The psychiatrist validates this impulse and then gently nudges Marina back to making contact with the feelings and to meta-awareness of them. This is what will eventually offer the holding that she desperately needs. As the poet Rumi said, "Open your hands if you want to be held."

The psychiatrist is teaching Marina how to recognize and accept various kinds of distressing inner experiences: thoughts, feelings, and even the urges "to do" something reactive. When Marina starts to overidentify with or to want to avoid any particular experience, he helps her reestablish the witnessing stance. Let's consider some of the implications of this move before we see what happens next for Marina.

Mindfulness of Thoughts Contributes to Psychological Flexibility and Rest

Mindfulness of thoughts is the recognition that thoughts are happening. Although it is easier to stay present to body sensations and emotions, when the mindfulness muscle is strengthened, or when we are reminded by a mindful listener, as Marina is in this dialogue, we find that it is possible to be meta-aware of thoughts as they occur in the present moment. If we have started to elaborate on the thoughts, the moment when we recognize that we have been swept away in them—for however long, or however far away they have taken us—is a moment of mindfulness. In a blink of time, we are right back in meta-awareness of the present moment, meta-aware that "thinking is like this." This will short-circuit the amplification that both immersing in and struggling with thoughts produce.

Thoughts and rules based on prior learning that are observed and whose content is no longer regarded as the only truth are less likely to influence the actions we take. We thereby obtain greater behavioral choice and are better able to act according to present values—that is, we gain more of the flexibility that is needed to cope with a crisis. By standing back and observing whatever arises in awareness, we also move from a fixed image of ourselves and the world toward a richer, more multifaceted landscape of existence. When we wake up from being lost in worries, there can be moments when we see the sunrays touching a leaf wavering in the wind and gain nourishing tastes of rest.

Mindfulness Curbs Experiential Avoidance of the Current Situation

If we expect mindfulness to deliver *only* blissful, serene, peaceful moments, we'll be disappointed. This expectation would imply that mindfulness may be pursued as yet another means by which to *avoid* experiencing inner pain and conflict. On the contrary, what we will experience is that mindfulness allows us to *know* and to *feel deeper* into the pain of the current situation.

Maurice's breaking into loud cries and weeping in Chapter 3 ("The ACT Model of Crisis Integration") is one example of this. The immensity of Maurice's loss was overwhelming to him at times. The exercise the psychiatrist suggested he deploy at such times was to alternate between feeling the pain and sensing his feet supported by the ground. Focusing attention on the feet is a way to reestablish an observer perspective and to nurture tranquility and rest. As we discuss further in Chapter 5, Maurice's cultivation of meta-awareness of his feet, with time, also increases his ability to offer meta-awareness to his pain. By staying with the mindfulness exercise, he will eventually learn how to move freely between leaning into *experiencing* the pain and leaning into *observing* the pain. In this practice, Maurice will experience that sometimes he is fully leaning into the pain and not at all into the observing mode, and sometimes vice versa. Other times, he may experience the pain and simultaneously witness it, a sort of 50/50 mode, which can also be 90/10, 40/60, or any ratio. Mindfully observing thus does not imply a mental gap between the meta-awareness of experience and the experience itself; rather, the mindfulness process and state are the foundation upon which you may place your trust as you incrementally open up and allow your entire heartbreak to be experienced—and held.

Experiential avoidance strategies not only take the shape of tangible distractions, such as screens or drugs. A more subtle and more pervasive phenomenon is avoidance in the form of thinking. The natural function of thinking is heavily biased toward figuring out ways, however intricate and complex, to either avoid danger or approach the desirable in the outside world. Likewise, thinking helps us avoid sensing what is going on inside our own skin. In other words, thoughts are often in the service of controlling other inner experiences, such as emotions: distracting from them, suppressing them, or reasoning with them to make them go away.

What then happens—when we let go of thinking thoughts, as happens in mindfulness—unwanted and unknown experiences arise, and that will feel uncomfortable, sometimes *very* uncomfortable. Not everyone who undertakes mindfulness is prepared for uncovering the deeper levels of pain from which our thought activity has attempted to distract us. The freedom and peace implicated in mindfulness do not mean freedom from unwanted inner experiences, only freedom from the need to struggle with them. Nevertheless, the emergence of these inner experiences will turn out to be a good thing.

In the dialogue with David in Chapter 3, for example, the psychiatrist reflected back David's thoughts about divorce and not wanting to be a burden in order to nurture his meta-awareness that they were just that— thoughts. She neither stayed on the level of thoughts nor engaged in dialogue with them. She labeled the thoughts as thoughts and acknowledged how painful it was to have thoughts like these. She then promptly moved on to the level of emotions and values. Moving beyond the thinking level opened up the possibility for David to feel deeper into the current situation and to understand it better.

The last bit of the dialogue with Marina touched on shame. This feeling was largely created by her and others' judgmental thoughts. It's an example of the way we evaluate our or others' lovability and acceptability in terms of static evaluations, such as *being* right or wrong, a winner or a loser, quick or slow, cute or ugly, smart or dumb, funny or boring, deserving or undeserving. Such evaluations and judgments, whether of others or of ourselves, are part of rule-based thinking and rarely provide us with any leverage to act in healthy ways.

If Marina were to remain mindful of her self-deprecating thoughts and the pervasive feelings of shame they produce, *other* feelings and unmet needs in her present situation might be able to surface. As the session with Marina continues, the psychiatrist brings her into contact with her inner life to see if she can establish a different kind of relationship with it.

Marina: Clinical Dialogue on Mindfulness and Acceptance of Present Feelings and Needs

Psychiatrist: You may stay with this as long as this shame needs, this wave of shame. Hold it in awareness, and when the wave has passed, you can go back and rest in awareness of your breath again.

Marina: (*Sits silent for a while, eyes still closed, staying with the process.*) I just feel so lonely. I don't know. Just so lonely. I have no one to turn to.

Psychiatrist: Yes, the infinite sense of loneliness, and the need to share your difficult reality with someone, someone who cares.

Marina: I long so much to lie in someone's arms and just rest. (*Tears begin to fall.*)

Psychiatrist: To rest in someone's loving and holding arms.

Marina: (*more tears*) I don't know if that is ever going to happen.

Psychiatrist: Yes, missing it so deeply.

Marina: I just want to be held by someone who knows—who knows and would still be willing to hold me. (*Tears keep flowing.*)

Psychiatrist: To be held and to know that this holding is for real. Of course.... A sense of honesty, maybe.

Marina: Yes, that would feel so nice. (*deep sigh*) I would be able to relax.

Psychiatrist: (*pause*) You want to love and be loved, to care and be cared for, to share your reality and your resting with someone, just like every other human being on this planet. Right now, we don't know in exactly what way you'll go out into the world and cultivate the love you want to give and the love you want to receive. What I suggest is

that you let that question rest for a little while. I believe that the way
will become clearer to you if you first practice relating to yourself in
a way that is more restful, tender, and caring.
Marina: That does sound logical to me. I actually feel calmer now than
I've done in a very long time.

The psychiatrist uses mindfulness and acceptance as a bridge to connect with Marina's deepest-held values and aspirations. From her loneliness and her unmet needs for holding and love, for honesty and shared
reality, for rest and calm, Marina will eventually move on and connect with
possibly the biggest pain of all—the prospect of missing out on having a
family. To allow all this to be felt, known, and accepted will take some time.
By cultivating her mindfulness skills, she will be able to give herself much
of the holding, knowing, honesty, and rest for which she yearns. Moreover,
shame-based self-appraisal and self-blaming cognition are in mindfulness
revealed for what they are and thus may be ameliorated (Boyd et al. 2018).
We bring Marina back in Chapter 6 to show how the psychiatrist helps her
foster self-forgiveness and self-compassion instead of self-criticism. All of
this pertains to her inner life; the next steps in her outer life have yet to be
discovered. Nevertheless, when Marina's perpetual thoughts and reactivity slow down, and she can recognize, name, and embrace her emotions,
needs, and values, she will be much more likely to make choices each step
of the way that bring healing to her situation.

To help Marina expand her mindfulness skills, she and the psychiatrist
agree that she will pay mindful attention to her breath for 15 minutes each
day. By bringing attention back, again and again, to present-moment experience, she will strengthen the mindfulness muscle so that each occasion she manages to bring mindful awareness to the present moment will
help her sustain the momentum—and so improve her ability to be mindful of the *next* upcoming moment. The psychiatrist also instructs Marina
to note any thoughts that hijack her attention to mindfulness of breath
and, afterward, to write them down and repeat them out loud, as fast as
she can, for 1 minute. This classic ACT intervention drives down the credibility of the negative thoughts, making them less enticing and less demanding of attention. To further cultivate her abilities, Marina agrees to do
a "mindfulness moment" five times a day during which she will scan her
inner world and notice any bodily sensations, feelings, thoughts, memories, or urges occurring in that moment.

It is worth mentioning here that a mustering of both courage and will
is often required the very moment we decide to move from thinking
thoughts to witnessing them because, as we've just seen, other painful experiences may show up. Moreover, we give a lot of credence to thoughts;

we commonly believe that we can figure things out through thinking. In reality, thinking rarely provides the new and creative ways of relating to ourselves and our situation that we need in crisis. Thoughts are largely based on previous learning and will provide solutions in line with that learning. What we can discover is that unexpected insights and possible solutions will surface when we let go into the present moment. As one of the most renowned thinkers of modern time, Albert Einstein, put it: "I think 99 times and find nothing. I stop thinking, swim in silence, and the truth comes to me."

Mindfulness Curbs Experiential Avoidance of Past Learning

The dialogue with Marina describes two benefits of mindfulness: its facilitation of psychological flexibility and rest and its capacity to curb experiential avoidance of the ongoing situation. A third benefit of moving from "avoidance by thinking thoughts" to "allowing by cultivating mindfulness" is that *past* experiences will be revealed. The inner experiences that arise in the present moment are in some way or other also composed by the past (Frith 2007). Whatever has come before—all we have learned through evolution, association, trial and error, models, and rules, all the momentum of our habits, memories, heartbreaks, losses, and traumas—will, with mindfulness, eventually surface in the present. The good news is that mindfulness simultaneously facilitates the equanimity and tenderness with which we can allow our afflictions from the recent or distant past to gradually become fully known and hence become susceptible to healing. Every time there is an instant or two of meta-awareness, the unfinished business of the heart gets an opportunity for resolution, and the charge of thoughts and urgent emotions relating to the past may thus be reduced.

Before we explore, in Chapter 5, more of why and how it is possible to transcend crises originating in the past as well as in the present, we need to consider the obvious question that comes up when individuals are invited to do the opposite of what they're used to doing—that is, to turn from avoidance to allowing: "Isn't this dangerous?" When experiences become known rather than suppressed, is there any risk of harm, of outcomes worse than would be expected in the absence of intervention (Dimidjian and Hollon 2010)? Could the surfacing of traumatic memories trigger a depressive episode? Could mindfulness exacerbate psychotic symptoms in individuals who are vulnerable to them? In short, does mindfulness raise any potential risks that we need to be alert to?

In intensive residential retreats, one meditates most of the day for a week or several weeks or even months. Observational studies of individuals undertaking such meditation schedules suggest that adverse events can occur, albeit infrequently (Creswell 2017). However, randomized controlled trials studying mindfulness-based clinical interventions involving smaller and spaced doses of mindfulness have revealed minimal risk of significant adverse events, such as impairment of mental health (Creswell 2017).

In this chapter, we concentrated on the cultivation of observant attitudes toward the skewed thought patterns prevalent in crises that can build up into anxiety, fatigue, and depression. In Chapter 5's exploration of the role of mindfulness of bodily sensations and emotion in crisis integration, we discuss how cumulative moments of exposure to painful emotions add up to produce positive momentum in the healing process. The gradual way in which mindfulness offers exposure may well be one reason why mindfulness-based interventions have significantly lower dropout rates among patients with PTSD than do trauma-focused therapies, while still being equally effective (Frost et al. 2014).

References

Allman JM, Watson KK, Tetreault NA, Hakeem AY: Intuition and autism: a possible role for Von Economo neurons. Trends Cogn Sci 9:367–73, 2005

Allman JM, Tetreault NA, Hakeem AY, et al: The von Economo neurons in frontoinsular and anterior cingulate cortex in great apes and humans. Brain Struct Funct 214:495–517, 2010

American Psychiatric Association: Diagnostic and Statistical Manual of Mental Disorders, 5th Edition, Text Revision. Washington, DC, American Psychiatric Association, 2022

Boyd JE, Lanius RA, McKinnon MC: Mindfulness-based treatments for posttraumatic stress disorder: a review of the treatment literature and neurobiological evidence. J Psychiatry Neurosci 43(1):7–25, 2018 29252162

Bruner E, Preuss TM, Chen X, Rilling JK: Evidence for expansion of the precuneus in human evolution. Brain Struct Funct 222:1053–60, 2017

Creswell JD: Mindfulness interventions. Annu Rev Psychol 68:491–516, 2017 27687118

Creswell JD, Lindsay EK: How does mindfulness training affect health? A mindfulness stress buffering account. Curr Dir Psychol Sci 23:401–407, 2014

Dimidjian S, Hollon SD: How would we know if psychotherapy were harmful? Am Psychol 65(1):21–33, 2010 20063907

Feinberg TE, Mallatt J: The nature of primary consciousness: a new synthesis. Conscious Cogn 43:113–127, 2016 27262691

Fleming SM, Daw ND: Self-evaluation of decision-making: a general Bayesian framework for metacognitive computation. Psychol Rev 124(1):91–114, 2017 28004960

Frith C, Dolan RJ: Brain mechanisms associated with top-down processes in perception. Philos Trans R Soc Lond B Biol Sci 352(1358):1221–1230, 1997 9304688

Frith CD: Making Up the Mind: How the Brain Creates Our Mental World. Oxford, UK, Blackwell, 2007

Frith CD: The neural basis of consciousness. Psychol Med 51(4):550–562, 2021 31481140

Frost ND, Laska KM, Wampold BE: The evidence for present-centered therapy as a treatment for posttraumatic stress disorder. J Trauma Stress 27(1):1–8, 2014 24515534

Goldstein J: Mindfulness: A Practical Guide to Awakening. Louisville, CO, Sounds True, 2013

Goldstein J: Knowing-loving-growing. Rickhanson.net, February 1, 2020. Available at: https://www.rickhanson.net/loving-knowing-and-growing-free-online-program. Accessed May 22, 2020.

James W: The Principles of Psychology. New York, Henry Holt, 1890

Kabat-Zinn J: Mindfulness-based interventions in context: past, present, and future. Clin Psychol Sci Pract 10:144–156, 2003

Kabat-Zinn J: Full Catastrophe Living: Using the Wisdom of Your Body and Mind to Face Stress, Pain, and Illness, Revised Edition. New York, Random House, 2013

Kabat-Zinn J: Wherever You Go, There You Are: Mindfulness Meditation for Everyday Life. London, Little, Brown, 2016

Kabat-Zinn J: The 20th Annual Dr. and Mrs. Frederick Barnes Lecture in Public Health, Featuring Jon Kabat-Zinn. Brown University, April 15, 2019. Available at: https://www.youtube.com/watch?v=kShpURJOpeE. Accessed April 26, 2021.

Kaas JH: The evolution of brains from early mammals to humans. Wiley Interdiscip Rev Cogn Sci 4:33-45, 2013

Kornfield J: The Art of Forgiveness, Lovingkindness, and Peace. New York, Bantam Books, 2008

Kornfield J: Awaken the one who knows. Jackkornfield.com, 2021. Available at: https://jackkornfield.com/awaken-one-knows. Accessed February 21, 2021.

Neff K: Self-compassion: an alternative conceptualization of a healthy attitude toward oneself. Self Ident 2:85–101, 2003

Polusny MA, Erbes CR, Thuras P, et al: Mindfulness-based stress reduction for posttraumatic stress disorder among veterans: a randomized clinical trial. JAMA 314(5):456–465, 2015 26241597

Salzburg S: Real Happiness: The Power of Meditation: A 28-Day Program. New York, Workman, 2011

Shea N, Frith CD: The Global Workspace Needs Metacognition. Trends Cogn Sci 23:560-71, 2019

Sumedho A: The Sound of Silence: The Ajahn Sumedho Anthology. Hemel Hempstead, UK, Amarawati Publications, 2014

Williams JM, Crane C, Barnhofer T, et al: Mindfulness-based cognitive therapy for preventing relapse in recurrent depression: a randomized dismantling trial. J Consult Clin Psychol 82(2):275–286, 2014 24294837

Wilson TD, Reinhard DA, Westgate EC, et al: Social psychology. Just think: the challenges of the disengaged mind. Science 345(6192):75–77, 2014 24994650

Yadavaia JE, Hayes SC, Vilardaga R: Using acceptance and commitment therapy to increase self-compassion: a randomized controlled trial. J Contextual Behav Sci 3:248-57, 2014

Young KS, van der Velden AM, Craske MG, et al: The impact of mindfulness-based interventions on brain activity: a systematic review of functional magnetic resonance imaging studies. Neurosci Biobehav Rev 84:424–433, 2018 28797556

5

Mindfulness of Body and Feeling

But deep in your body,
your force and your fears
live united, heart and hand,
within an all-encompassing
Arc of And.

—Elizabeth English (2023)

Bringing in the Body in Crisis Integration

Judging by how little emphasis conventional psychiatry and psychology place on the ability to sense the body from within in the context of dealing with suffering, it seems as though we are still living within the paradigm of René Descartes, at least in the West. Descartes was the 17th-century French philosopher who singled out the mind as something non-material and, as such, fundamentally distinct from the body. Many contemporary psychological interventions overlook the body in their focus on the triad of thought, feeling, and behavior. Although psychiatry today is inarguably based on biology, clinical practice does not typically emphasize patients' experience of their body from within.

Where did the body go? Whatever the answer, mindfulness of body is at the heart of the ACT model of crisis integration. Many psychiatric disorders—including mood and anxiety disorders, PTSD, OCD, personality disorders, psychotic disorders, substance use disorders, and other chronic conditions—have one thing in common: dysfunction in correctly evaluating internal bodily states (Barrett and Simmons 2015; Khalsa et al. 2018;

Löffler et al. 2018; Paulus and Stein 2010; Paulus et al. 2019; Smith et al. 2020, 2021; Yoris et al. 2017). Because one of the brain's primary functions is to develop accurate models of the world and the body in order to facilitate conditions that are ideal for the organism's functioning, this should not come as a surprise.

In acute crisis, emotions may be intense, the shock surreal, and the bodily stress reactions overwhelming. Maurice, whom we met in Chapter 3 ("The ACT Model of Crisis Integration"), provides a strong example of this acute disheartenment, having traumatically lost his partner and newborn child. In prolonged crisis, it is common for most of those responses of body and emotion to have gone into hiding and to reveal themselves only occasionally—and confusingly, because they often do so without much warning. In this chapter we meet Lucía, who suffered abuse and neglect throughout her childhood and thus, as a survival mechanism, has closed off from her inner bodily and emotional experiences—a behavior pattern the ACT model describes as *experiential avoidance*. As an adult, she has not yet learned how to feel whole and alive again, and she experiences suicidal thoughts. As we saw in the dialogues with Maurice in Chapter 3 and Marina in Chapter 4 ("A Field Guide to Mindfulness"), mindfulness is both restful and revealing in crisis. It is restful in that it provides a tranquil refuge in which to soothe oneself and a pause from thinking the unruly thoughts that arise from efforts to avoid or cling to unpleasant and pleasant experiences, together with justifications of these efforts. It is revealing because repressed bodily and emotional responses to current or past situations will gradually surface to be experienced. In crisis, bodily responses and emotions tend to be either in uproar or silenced. Tender guidance is therefore required when a patient undertakes to discover, receive, accept, and embrace them, as we illustrate in a case study later in this chapter.

If you ask patients exactly where their emotions are located, you're likely to elicit a baffled response. Psychiatrists also may not be able to answer this question as it pertains to their own emotional experience. Feelings are generally seen as just being there. Even after some introspection, the common conceptualization of emotions is that they are situated somewhere around us, such as in front of the head or torso. However, to move from avoidance to awareness of emotions in crisis, it is helpful to know a bit more precisely where to start looking.

This chapter is built on two main propositions. First, that emotions are closely linked to the brain's processing of the body's internal states. Second, that how we relate to these bodily states will determine whether, in crisis, we will experience more and prolonged suffering or a gradual increase of well-being. According to the ACT model of crisis, any sustained avoidance, distraction, or controlling of bodily sensations and correlated emotions will intensify the crisis. In contrast, the more equanimity, acceptance, and awareness we maintain with respect to our body's internal states, the further we will go in integrating the crisis.

Several of the clinical case studies we present in this book make use of the faculty of sensing the body from within. Chapter 4 describes a few of the many purposes this clinical tool serves (Figure 5–1). It brings the patient back to the present moment—the first dimension of mindfulness. It supports meta-awareness of what is going on in the present moment—the second dimension of mindfulness. Further down the line, it supports meta-awareness of any aversion to or desiring of present-moment experience—the third dimension of mindfulness. It defuses the impetus to elaborate one's thoughts—the tendency of thoughts to generate further thoughts and feelings—and impedes avoidance of underlying feelings and needs. It also provides a place to rest one's attention and a way to recharge and soothe oneself in times of distress.

In this chapter, we explore in detail how mindfulness of body can facilitate crisis integration: how it can be used to reveal and integrate bodily and emotional responses to present and past events, increase so-called distress tolerance, reduce habitual responses based on prior learning, improve accurate knowing of body and emotion, improve homeostatic regulation, deepen one's trust that one's body is a safe place in which to live, and enhance one's agency and one's presence to "what is." To understand the whys and wherefores of all this, we need first to examine how the brain goes about the tasks of perceiving "what's out there"—or *exteroception*—and, especially relevant to mindfulness of body and emotion, of perceiving "what's in there"—*interoception*.

Our examination includes the unlikely story of how Thomas Bayes, an eighteenth-century English minister, has become a celebrity of twenty-first century neuroscience. His simple mathematical algorithm can be used to explain how the neural system predicts, perceives, and learns about our ever-changing bodily and emotional states (Fletcher and Frith 2009; Friston 2020).

Interoception: Sensing the Body From Within

The concept of interoception was coined in the early 1900s to refer to the perception of the body from within (Sherrington 1906), the sense of a

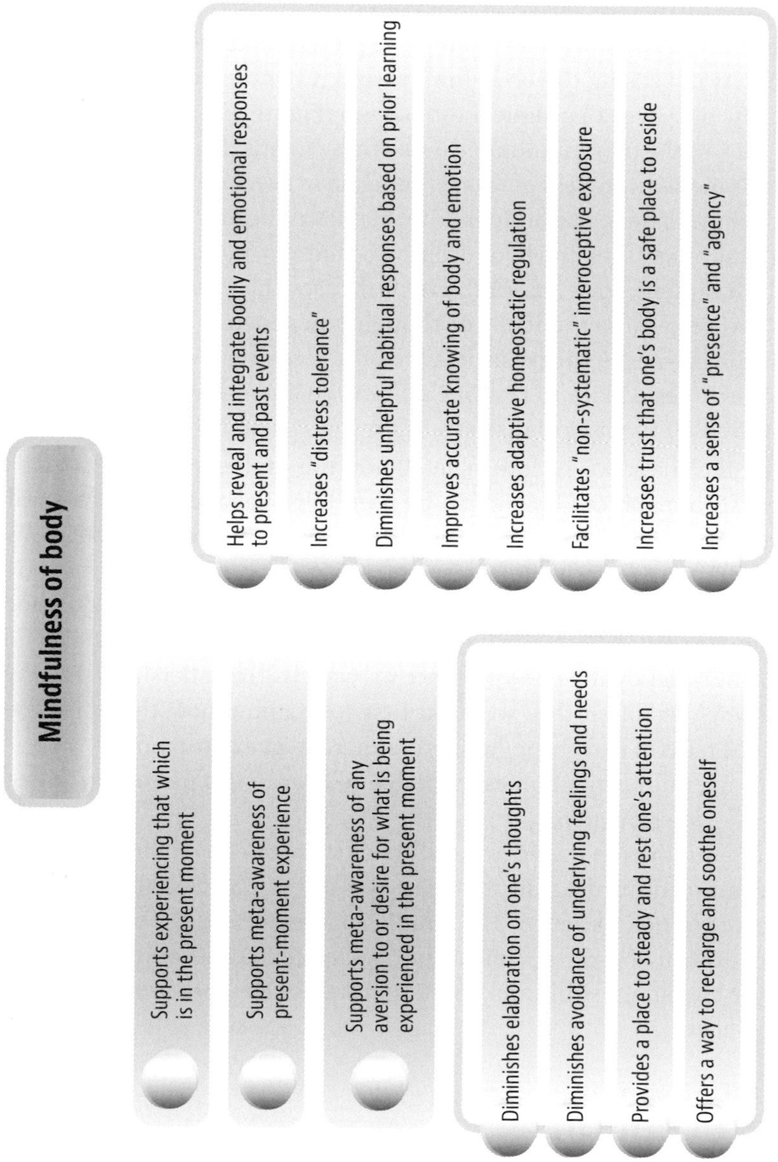

Mindfulness of body

Supports experiencing that which is in the present moment

Supports meta-awareness of present-moment experience

Supports meta-awareness of any aversion to or desire for what is being experienced in the present moment

Diminishes elaboration on one's thoughts

Diminishes avoidance of underlying feelings and needs

Provides a place to steady and rest one's attention

Offers a way to recharge and soothe oneself

Helps reveal and integrate bodily and emotional responses to present and past events

Increases "distress tolerance"

Diminishes unhelpful habitual responses based on prior learning

Improves accurate knowing of body and emotion

Increases adaptive homeostatic regulation

Facilitates "non-systematic" interoceptive exposure

Increases trust that one's body is a safe place to reside

Increases a sense of "presence" and "agency"

Figure 5–1.   Functions of mindfulness of body as a clinical tool.

"material me" (Craig 2003). It is distinct from the perception of the external environment through sight, hearing, touch, smell, and taste, called exteroception, as well as the sense of the body's position and movements, or proprioception (Sherrington 1906). Today, interoception is defined a bit more stringently as the nervous system's perception and integration of signals originating from within the body, thereby providing a momentary mapping of the body's internal landscape (Craig 2002, 2009; Khalsa et al. 2018). Interoception can be both *unaware*, involving neural activity on lower levels such as the spinal cord, and *aware*, in relation to higher-order neural processing in the brain's cortex. Moment-by-moment interoceptive mapping is necessary because the inner and external worlds of the body's physiological conditions are in constant flux. In order to prompt adaptive responses, the nervous system closely monitors any possible change inside and outside the organism. The maintenance of desired physiological states, known as *homeostasis*, is critical to the survival of all living creatures (Cannon 1932).

We saw in Chapter 4 that *aware* perception of the body from within— a subjective interoceptive experience—relates to a primary type of consciousness that we call "sentience." *Meta-awareness* of this interoceptive experience is awareness of having such an aware subjective experience; it's a secondary type of consciousness. Whereas interoception equates to sensing the body from within, meta-awareness has a witnessing stance *toward* these sensations. In this chapter, we further unpack the conceptual and experiential distinction between interoception and meta-awareness of interoceptive information.

How Does Interoception Relate to Emotion and Feeling?

At the basic biological level, it is easy to see how homeostasis becomes the basis for the feelings we experience. When the osmotic pressure of sodium increases, we feel thirsty. When blood sugar level drops, we feel hungry. When body temperature falls, we feel cold. These "homeostatic emotions" motivate behaviors aimed to maintain the body's ideal state: drinking, eating, putting on warmer clothes (Craig 2003; Gizowski and Bourque 2018). The sense of disrupted homeostasis produces the inclination to reestablish balance.

Sitting at the interface between the inner and outer worlds of the body, the brain samples both interoceptive and exteroceptive information (Paulus et al. 2019). In addition to disrupted homeostasis, emotions can be triggered by environmental stimuli signaling danger or opportunity—that is, stimuli with an *aversive* or *appetitive* quality. Such stimuli elicit core emotions such as fear, anger, and joy and activate capacities to move us away from or toward the stimuli in question. Here, too, the body is involved. When you feel fear in the proximity of danger, your heart and breathing rates increase, blood is directed from your stomach to your muscles, and so on. What may be surprising is that interoception is the foundation of the neural encoding of all feelings, including the more complex and subtle ones (Craig 2009).

Seen through the lens of evolution, emotions—whether prompted internally or externally—help the organism to stay alive and thrive (Damasio 1994). *Emotion* can be defined in various ways. From the perspective of evolutionary psychology, emotion is considered to comprise physiological, expressive, and experiential components (Dolan 2002; Lane and Schwartz 1987). Just as perception and behavior can be processed without awareness, so can emotion (Carlsson et al. 2004; Öhman and Soares 1994; Öhman et al. 2007), although it is more automatic and imprecise. Fully experienced emotions, on the other hand, increase the flexibility of the response and the likelihood of choosing an appropriate action (Lane and Schwartz 1987). For present purposes, we view emotion as comprising a bodily response, a motivation toward action, and a subjective experience of the emotion—or what in everyday speech are called "feelings."

Awareness of what is happening in our body is crucial to being in tune with our feelings, which in turn promotes general well-being and appropriate responses to challenges from the world. James Joyce's (1914) line "Mr. Duffy lived a short distance from his body" gives a precise image of a person out of sync with himself and his surroundings.

Anterior Insula: The Hub in the Neural Network Encoding Both Interoception and Feelings

The *insula*, Latin for "island," is the brain's fifth lobe. It is not visible from a surface view of the brain (Figure 5–2), tucked beneath the overlap of the temporal and frontal cortices, and is among the cortical regions most expanded in humans compared with the corresponding regions in other primates (Bauernfeind et al. 2013). The insula is a critical neural substrate for both interoception and feelings, which accentuates just how interrelated these experiences are (Craig 2014; Gu et al. 2013).

Around the turn of the new millennium, the afferent neural pathways carrying information about the body's physiological status became more fully known (Craig 2002). Neural routes that provide information about the entire body—including the cardiovascular, pulmonary, gastrointesti-

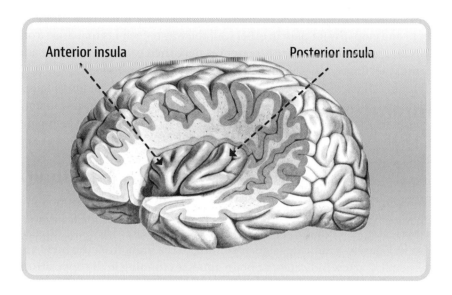

Figure 5–2. **The insula.**

nal, genitourinary, nociceptive, chemosensory, osmotic, thermoregulatory, visceral, immune, and autonomic systems *and* the skin, joints, and muscles—were then described all the way up to the posterior part of the insula (summarized in Khalsa et al. 2018).

Much of the body's homeostatic regulation happens either locally at the cellular level or farther up at the level of the spinal cord, brainstem, or subcortical nuclei. Information about any remaining imbalances in the body's condition that reaches the brain will have its primary cortical representation in the insula. In this way, the posterior insula is like a "captive audience" for interoceptive information from the body (Damasio 1994).

The mapping of the interoceptive signals propagates from the posterior to the anterior insula, the anterior part encoding more complex and abstract information. In the anterior insula, information from sensory afferent nerves from the body becomes integrated with contextual information to produce subjective emotional experience (Craig 2009). The anterior insula is well situated for this job, having widespread bidirectional connectivity to the cortex's other four lobes and to subcortical structures such as the amygdala, brainstem, thalamus, and basal ganglia (Flynn 1999). The insula is thus the neural network's hub not only for the "body in the mind" but also for feelings.

Neuroimaging studies show activity in the anterior insula during the subjective experience of basic emotions, such as anger, fear, happiness, and sadness; complex ones, such as lust, uncertainty, unfairness, indignation, and empathy for pain in others; all the way to feelings that arise from listening to music. All these experiences have their own interoceptive and contextual fingerprint (Craig 2009; Singer et al. 2004, 2009).

Interoception and Feeling Based on Prior Knowledge and Present Events

The feedforward of sensory signals from the body to the brain for registration, integration, and response is far from being the whole story. Our experience of the body in the present moment comes as much, if not more, from the brain's guesses about our bodily state based on previous experiences as it does from the state of the body itself. The ascending arrow in Figure 5–3 indicates signals coming to the brain from the body; the descending arrow indicates the brain's guesses running in the opposite direction, from the brain to the body (von Helmholtz 1866/1962). The brain uses prior knowledge to predict what signals it should be receiving and what they should signify and compares these with the actual signals of present events. In other words, interoception depends on comparisons of *descending predictions* of the internal bodily state and *ascending signals* of the actual state. Our experience of interoception, and indeed exteroception, does not equate to what we sense directly but is a computational compromise between our expectation of what we think we should be sensing and the actual sensory input.

In other words, we literally predict our way into our sense of embodied experience and our emotions, based on our previous experiences. One key premise of the ACT approach is that excessive reliance on prior knowledge when we evaluate a situation and choose actions produces psychological rigidity, which may instigate crises and so perpetuate suffering. The corollary is that updating our knowledge, revisiting our values, and broadening our repertoire of strategies facilitate the psychological flexibility that is key to our well-being. In other words, overdependence on prior internal models of bodily states instigates crisis, and the remedy is found in updated models of inner experience generated through mindfulness of body. Let us unpack first what is meant by the idea of the brain as a prediction generator.

Prediction—the Brain's Way of Getting Ahead

One thing that *all* the brain's learning systems have in common is that they all involve making and updating predictions, continuously and often without awareness. As Lisa Feldman Barrett remarked, "our brains didn't

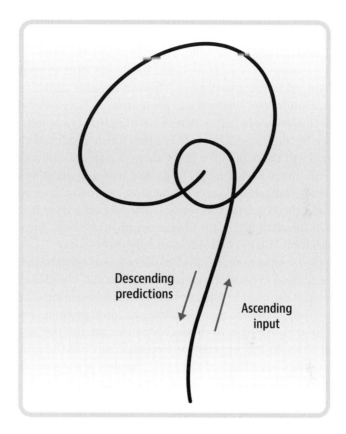

Descending
predictions

Ascending
input

Figure 5–3. **Interoception, a computational compromise between signals the brain predicts it will receive from the body and those it actually receives.**

evolve to react to the world around us, but rather to predict what's going to happen to us next" (Armstrong 2019). When you see a snake, you don't have to pick it up to figure out whether it is poisonous. We *predict* that the snake is dangerous because our forerunners who predicted this danger were able to survive and passed on this knowledge through phylogenesis. In Chapter 2, "The ACT Model of Crisis Instigation," we called this type of learning "evolutionary-shaped learning." Through verbal model-based learning, too, we predict and update predictions of which approaches and situations will be good for us and which will be bad. For example, "If I perform well, I *predict* that I will be loved and included in the social group." Prediction is even central to the most basic Pavlovian associations, such as when the perception of the sound of a bell causes salivation. The term *associative learning* is misleading here because the mere juxtaposition of a bell and food in time is not sufficient to cause any learning.

In one experiment, Pavlov reported that even after 374 pairings of a bell and food, no learning took place. This was because the bell was always rung 5–10 seconds *after* the food was presented. To have an effect, a stimulus needs to act as a prediction that something that is wanted (or feared) will happen in the future. Only if it has previously predicted the appearance of food will the sound of a bell induce the autonomic reflex of salivation (Frith 2007; Pavlov 1927). Pavlovian learning about rewards and punishments establishes a direct connection between the neutral stimulus (bell) and the response (salivation). The response does not therefore require an internal model of the phenomenon of the bell's previous association with food; it is elicited automatically (Frith 2021).

Perception, on the other hand, *does* make use of models. In Chapters 2 and 3 we described in detail the verbal kind of model-based learning. This chapter focuses on another aspect of model-based learning that relates to perception and, in particular, as it relates to interoception. The purpose of model-based learning is to choose responses predicting the most beneficial outcomes for the organism on a reliable basis. In the course of this, perception generates models of the world; models of the present situation are compared with models of past situations, and responses are chosen based on outcomes of past situations (Frith 2021).

As we reviewed in Chapter 4, the model-based system relates to sentience, the brain's capacity to create an internal experience of external objects and of the body. This system is thought to have evolved on top of the earlier, model-free learning system. It thereby has freed organisms to respond more flexibly than when they only respond to their environment automatically. The system enabling metacognition and meta-awareness in humans then evolved on top of the model-based system (see Figure 4–1), freeing us from subservience to our models of the world (Frith 2021) and so granting us yet more psychological flexibility. The three dimensions of mindfulness described in Chapter 4–1) experiencing that which is in the present moment, 2) having meta-awareness of present-moment experience, and 3) having meta-awareness of any aversion to or desire for what is being experienced in the present moment—use the model-based system together with the capacities for metacognition and meta-awareness.

From an evolutionary perspective, organisms accessed evolutionary-shaped learning first, then model-free learning, then nonverbal and verbal model-based learning, then metacognition and meta-awareness. This line of development brought increasing flexibility along the gradient from lower-

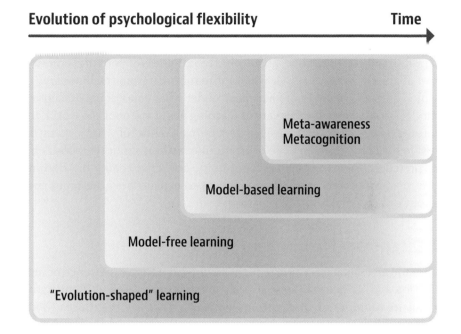

Figure 5–4. **Evolution of the neural system's learning systems.**

to higher-order nervous systems. The human neural system, being of the highest order, gives access to all these forms of learning (see Figure 5–4).

Broadly speaking, the learning systems are implemented in different neural structures: model-free learning about rewards and punishments uses subcortical areas of the brain, and perceptual model-based learning about states of the world uses a frontoparietal network together with the specific cortical areas that process information relating to sight, hearing, taste, smell, and bodily sensations. Just as the visual cortex, for example, is implied in model-based learning about what we see, the insula encodes bodily sensations and related emotions. How metacognition and meta-awareness map onto the underlying brain activity is not precisely known, but a few higher-order brain regions are certainly involved, such as the cingulate cortex; the prefrontal cortex, including the frontopolar cortex, an area right behind the forehead; and the precuneus (Frith 2021). Certainly, the specific brain area encoding whatever one's mindful attention is directed toward will also be active. Mindfulness of body, for example, activates the insula. What's more, mindfulness training has been shown to increase the ability to pay attention to body sensation, producing greater functional activity and cortical thickness in the insula than in people with no such training (Farb et al. 2007, 2013; Tang et al. 2015).

If we are curious about the brain's processing of interoception and emotion and, down the line, about what mindfulness of body and emotion can do for us during crisis, we will want to move on from the blobology of which areas of the brain are activated under what conditions. Perceptual model-based learning takes care of learning about states of the world. Interoception, in particular, involves generating a model of what is going on inside the body, through which current information about the body is interpreted. In the neuroscience community, *predictive coding* has become the most widespread and popular theory to explain how the brain goes about this task (Friston 2020; Friston et al. 2010).

Perception Through Predictive Coding

To build an explanatory bridge between the subjective experience of perception and its neurobiological basis, neuroscience tries to identify the requisite computational steps, or algorithms, that the brain uses (Marr 1982; Smith et al. 2021). This is where Thomas Bayes comes in. Three hundred years ago, Bayes presented a mathematical theorem that has recently been dusted off and proven useful in diverse scientific disciplines, most notably in epidemiology and neuroscience. His algorithm's broad usefulness hinges on the fact that it generates the probability for certain things to happen, and the probable cause behind what is happening, using the previously known probability and the possible cause of other, related things, happening (Bayes 1763).

The explanation of perception in terms of predictive coding can be seen as likening the brain to a little scientist who actively generates predictions and explanations of the stimuli they encounter as, in effect, hypotheses tested against direct sensory evidence (Seth and Friston 2016). In other words, everything we perceive is filtered by and understood through prior knowledge.

The key concept in Bayes' algorithm is "the probable *cause behind* what is happening." In visual perception, for example, the brain receives two-dimensional information from the eye's retina about different intensities and frequencies of light—the retina being a neural array, more or less flat, situated at one point in space at one point in time. Our three-dimensional experience of shapes, forms, location, and colors is created by the brain through inferences about the "causes behind" the information coming from the eyes. In a similar way, every sensory experience is constructed by the brain on the basis of prior knowledge, just as much as it is by present events. What we perceive in the moment is in large part a reflection of what our brain predicts is happening on the basis of previous experiences.

When it comes to the body, neither a perception of the shape and location of the internal organs nor the exact body temperature, pulse rate, or osmotic pressure is of much everyday use. What is vital, however, is to be updated about the body's internal condition and homeostasis. It has been suggested that, in the case of interoceptive information, the "probable cause behind what is happening" is experienced as emotions (Barrett and Simmons 2015; Seth 2013; Seth and Friston 2016). To give two simple examples: increased heartbeat may be experienced as fear, and increased osmotic pressure causes the homeostatic emotion of thirst. From the perspective of predictive coding, emotional experiences are thus not fundamentally different from experiences of sensory perception, such as the visual recognition that a tree trunk is cylindrical and not flat.

We may be forgiven if we don't have the mathematical acumen to grasp the full intricacy and implications of Bayes' algorithm. Nevertheless, much will be gained if we understand even a small portion of it, because predictive coding has gained a great deal of empirical support in the field of perception, including interoception and emotion (Barrett and Simmons 2015; Seth 2013; Seth and Friston 2016) and mindfulness of body (Farb et al. 2015). It is furthermore considered to provide a better understanding of many sorts of mental suffering (Paulus et al. 2019), ranging from schizophrenia (Fletcher and Frith 2009; Friston 2020) to autism (Palmer et al. 2015) and affective disorders (Barrett and Simmons 2015; Clark et al. 2018).

Prediction Error: Mismatch Between Prior Knowledge and Present Events

By framing perception as a learning system, we have already implied its inherent potential for updating and calibration. In a world of change, predictions based on prior knowledge will not always match what is going on in the present. When there is a discrepancy between what is predicted and what is actually happening, an ascending signal will convey this information from the lower processing level to a higher one—that is, up the hierarchy of the nervous system. In the case of interoception, the perceptual process will involve descending predictions about internal bodily states and counterflowing ascending interoceptive signals (see Figure 5-3).

Predictive coding is in this way implemented according to a hierarchical design. Top-down neural connections transfer predictions based on models from higher processing levels to lower ones. Building models of the world through predictive coding is a routine part of the perception process not only in the brain but in the nervous system as a whole. The integration of the top-down predictions and bottom-up input hence takes place not only on aware levels of information processing but also on un-aware lower levels of the nervous system. In the case of vision, for exam-ple, the visual cortex takes care of high-level processing of vision and the retina the lowest level.

For interoception, the insula is part of the highest level of the process-ing hierarchy; the neurons innervating the bodily organs are on the lowest level, and there are numerous other processing levels in-between, such as the brainstem and spinal cord. Interoceptive predictive coding thus does not take place only on the cortical level; it involves many crosswalks be-tween predictions descending from above and sensory input ascending from below.

It follows that inferences about the probable causes of events made ac-cording to Bayes' theorem should be understood not only as consciously held beliefs but as neuronally encoded probability distributions. They are sometimes called "Bayesian beliefs" about the causes of sensory signals, but for simplicity we refer to them here mainly as "prior knowledge" or "models" and occasionally as "beliefs." All of these concepts refer to prior knowledge sustained by the neural system.

An experience that does not challenge the descending predictions is, in effect, predictable, and thus is less likely to be attended to, if not com-pletely ignored. When a mismatch occurs, however, between what the brain expects and what it gets, a *prediction error* arises (Seth 2018). This prediction error alerts the brain that its current model is slightly wrong and that something in the world, whether outside or inside the body, ap-pears to have changed. This is a problem the brain will aim to resolve.

Prediction Errors Resolved by Changing the World or Changing the Model

There are two principal ways in which a prediction error can be resolved. The first of these has implications for one's sense of *agency*, and the sec-ond has implications for mindfulness of body and one's sense of *presence* (Farb et al. 2015).

Seeking or Changing the Evidence to Accord With What One Already Believes

Actions can be taken so that sensory samples are selected or even changed to better fit the model. This contributes to stable models and obviates the need to process all the sensations coming in from the outer world. The chief disadvantage of this solution is inflexibility (Fletcher and Frith 2009). Unchallenged models become strong and can lead to the downplaying or even ignoring of important changes and experiences.

Learning Without a Teacher

The prediction error can be used to update the model into one that better corresponds to the world. On *short* timescales, this corresponds to perception itself—a reminder that perception is not merely a passive readout of input (von Helmholtz 1866/1962)—and happens when the prediction error is considered valid enough to update the perceptual guesses. Instead of being disregarded as predicted, the ascending information updates the prediction, which results in a perceptual experience. On *longer* timescales, such updating of prior knowledge corresponds to what we know as learning about the world (Smith et al. 2019). Learning happens when something significant is not fully accounted for by the prediction, and the current evidence is used to update the model (Frith 2007).

In the first way of resolving prediction errors, the model changes the world as it is perceived; in the second, the world changes the model. The combination of the two underlines the strong continuity between prediction based on prior learning, perception, and learning from present evidence (Seth 2013). For interoception, remember, "the world" equals the inner world of the body.

Before we explore further the two principal ways in which prediction errors are resolved, let's consider *which* prediction errors will be taken into account. In determining what impact to give a prediction error relative to a model, the neural system considers both the magnitude and the reliability afforded to the prediction error. We may imagine the neural system utilizing what in statistical terms are called the *mean* (i.e., magnitude) and the *standard deviation* (i.e., inferred validity or "precision") when it is determining whether a prediction error can be brushed aside or should have an effect upon perception and learning. It is logical that a prediction error with low magnitude and low precision would be more likely to be disregarded than one with high magnitude and high precision.

A mutual interaction occurs between the precision of the prediction errors and the precision of the prior belief. Typically, when the precision of the prediction error is low, the precision of the belief will be high, and vice versa. This effect propagates up the hierarchy because a prior belief becomes the evidence for the prediction error at the next level up.

Interoception and Feeling Through Predictive Coding

Interoceptive prediction errors insufficiently resolved at lower processing levels are passed up the hierarchy—for interoception, to the posterior insula—and even farther up to the anterior insula for emotional processing, thus giving rise to subjective feeling experience (Seth and Friston 2016). In other words, interoceptive prediction errors detected by the posterior insula, via iterative comparison of the brain's expectation of bodily information with the actual incoming bodily information, are forwarded up one more level in the hierarchy to the anterior insula. Emotions are the result of the integration of these ascending prediction errors and predictions based on prior knowledge (Gu et al. 2013; Seth and Friston 2016).

A feeling can be of the most basic kind, such as the sense of whether what's happening is good or bad, pleasant or unpleasant, thus ascribing appetitive or aversive value to an inner or outer event. The feeling can also be more complex and nuanced, as when present events are integrated with diversified prior and contextual knowledge.

No brain area functions in isolation. Other parts of the brain help the insula infer the likely internal and external causes of changes in the body's physiological condition. Nevertheless, the insula plays a crucial role in supporting interoception and bodily self-representation, as well as one's emotional state, including the subjective experience of feeling (Craig 2009; Critchley and Harrison 2013; Gu et al. 2013).

What's more, the insula also provides descending interoceptive predictions that drive the autonomic nervous system (as well as the endocrine and immune responses), not only to predict but also to generate future bodily states, as in "changing the world (i.e., the body) to fit the model" (Critchley and Garfinkel 2017). In such ways, the insula both *responds to* and *influences* the body's homeostasis.

Interoceptive Prediction Errors Resolved by Adjusting the Body or the Model

We have seen that the prediction error in perception can be resolved by adjusting either the world as it is perceived to fit the model or the model to fit the world. Since "the world" in interoception equates to the inner world of the body, the interoceptive prediction error can be resolved either by changing the body to fit the model or by changing the model to fit the body. Both options are adaptive in their own way, and both are needed to enable flexible and adaptive responses to external or internal disruptions. However, excessive "adjusting the body to fit the model" can lead to suffering, as we unpack later in the section "Crisis Instigation With Interoceptive Avoidance." Fortunately, this suffering can be reversed by adjusting the model to fit the body through mindfulness of body.

One example of adjusting the body to fit the model is when there is a discrepancy between an expected state of calm (model) and an accelerating heart rate (body). One appropriate response could be, "I sense an increased heartbeat, I feel afraid, and I know there is good reason to be afraid here. I'll get away from here to a place where I'll be safe again." Here the body is adjusted to the model of calm through overt action. Another example is the act of drinking a glass of water when you're thirsty. Drinking the water changes the physiological state to conform more closely with homeostatic expectation of an optimal osmotic pressure, which is a favorable model of one aspect of the body's inner state.

These two examples also clarify that a mismatch—a prediction error—between the expected and the observed states generates a *perception of a bodily state*, a *subjective experience of emotion*, and a *motivation to resolve the prediction error*. These correspond to the three aspects of emotion referred to earlier in this chapter. The resolving, or at least minimizing, of the prediction error requires one to adjust the physiological state to bring it in alignment with a predicted model of the body.

Important to both adaptive and maladaptive functioning is that not all adjustment of the body to fit the model involves overt skeletomuscular behavior. For one thing, the response can include a covert shifting of attention to sensory information that will affirm the belief. Adjustment of the body can also build on the autonomic nervous system's top-down regulation of physiology. This latter type of interoceptive regulation largely happens automatically and outside awareness. Only when stressors exceed one's autonomic regulatory capacity will ascending prediction errors reach the cortex for conscious processing and motivate adaptive interaction with the environment (Seth 2013). The ensuing action, if successful, promotes a sense of agency or confidence in one's ability to change bodily states in a desired direction. The common denominator of both overt and covert actions is the aim to reduce the prediction error by changing the body sensations to fit the prior expectation.

One example of adjusting the model to fit the body is when I perceive an accelerating heartbeat (body) when I would rather feel calm (model). Because I'm in a safe situation, as far as I know, I don't have to do anything. I can witness the heartbeat and accept that it's okay. This particular situation could pertain to Kai, whom we met in Chapter 2, who experiences mounting anxiety when approaching a bus he is supposed to be taking.

Here the functional resolving, or minimizing, of the prediction error hinges on updating one's beliefs about the bodily sensations in such a way as to broaden the tolerable range of pulse rate. The second half of this chapter reveals more about why mindfulness of body in this situation will make it easier for someone to accept heart palpitations in the future and thus move on with what they really need to be doing.

The ability to minimize prediction errors is foundational for health and well-being. Ultimately, this ability demands a balance between "adjusting the body to fit the model" and "adjusting the model to fit the body." Adjusting the body corresponds in psychological terms to a sense of *agency*— one's ability to effect positive changes in bodily states. Adjusting the model corresponds to *presence*, or *being present*, one's aware perception of what is going on in the moment (Farb et al. 2015). Agency relates to engagement and mindful doing in the ACT model, and presence is linked to acceptance and mindful being. Agency, engagement, and mindful doing, together with presence, acceptance, and mindful being, will support a person's regulatory flexibility in response to change. Successful reduction of interoceptive prediction errors by means of either agency or presence facilitates homeostatic balance in the organism as a whole. During crisis instigation, however, this adaptive adjustment can break down in several ways.

Crisis Instigation With Interoceptive Avoidance

The predictive coding model of interoception sheds light on why avoidance of bodily sensations can instigate crisis and why mindfulness of body can integrate the crisis. By conceptualizing the brain as a prediction generator, we can understand the bodily sensations experienced in the present moment as reflecting not only incoming bodily signals but also the brain's predictions, based on previous experience, of what is going on inside the body.

If the brain treats prediction error signals from the body as unreliable or even unwanted indicators of present bodily states, it will end up with interoception that is primarily determined by prior knowledge (Smith et al. 2020). Such aberrant updating of the internal model of the body will lead to long-term failure to *correctly* interpret the "material me." In many psychiatric conditions, a largely overlooked contributor to disability and suffering is the patient's continuous misestimation of the internal state of their body, which in turn impairs their ability to correctly understand their feelings and to interact effectively with their environment (Barrett and Simmons 2015; Khalsa et al. 2018; Lane et al. 2015; Löffler et al. 2018; Paulus et al. 2019; Seth 2013; Smith et al. 2018, 2021; Yoris et al. 2017).

In the language of predictive coding, this misestimation transpires through *overweighting* the validity of prior knowledge relative to prediction errors or *underweighting* the validity of prediction errors relative to the prior model. Both tendencies result in a diminished level of interoceptive awareness and hence impair one's ability to recognize and understand one's own emotions.

A brain uninclined to update its models of the body will also have difficulty keeping the body's physiological conditions within their optimum homeostatic ranges, something normally achieved through behavioral adjustments (Barrett and Simmons 2015). When we are oblivious of the signals regarding our body's basic needs, we are less likely to take actions that are beneficial for our body. A continuous failure to sustain homeostasis will lead, over time, to the accumulation of deleterious physiological consequences (McEwen and Stellar 1993; Sterling 2014) that may instigate crises.

This is where mindfulness of body comes in as a powerful tool to turn the situation around. Increasing attunement to subtle or not-so-subtle bodily cues will lead to more insight into one's feelings, needs, and values and to a better ability to choose appropriate responses. To understand how this works in practice, it will be helpful to explore a few different ways that poor body perception comes about.

Experiential Avoidance of Present Bodily Events

The essence of a crisis situation is that it is experienced at the bodily level as overpowering, overwhelming, and unbearable. The stress commonly exceeds *both* the covert autonomic regulatory capacity and the overt behavioral options to alleviate the stress response. In other words, there are no responses available to sufficiently resolve the interoceptive prediction error, and this results in an assault on the sense of agency. Nothing the person does seems to help promote bodily ease.

Moreover, the existing bodily sensations are usually perceived as too intense to continue to experience, witness, and know, thus violating the capacity to be present to what is going on inside. A sense of powerlessness and feeling overwhelmed can break in, such that ascending interoceptive prediction errors become associated with danger and threat. Associations with danger that arise during shocking or painful events can involve both model-based and model-free learning. Just as Pavlov's dog acquired a salivatory response to the bell and did not require a conscious model of food, bell, salivation, and their internal associations (Pavlov 1927), so does much of our own learning happen without our awareness, or "preconsciously" (Frith 2021). Parts of our knowing of the threatening situation may thus not initially be accessible to concepts or words; what is left to be experienced is the intense bodily response of discomfort, urge, and panic. The strategy commonly used in such circumstances is to avoid, inhibit, and, if necessary, dissociate from interoceptive signals, especially in the case of traumatic events.

Even though avoidance of sensory signals may be the only response available at the time of an overwhelming event, trouble awaits if bodily and emotional avoidance of this sort lingers over time. When the terrifying outer situation becomes history, the most frightening phenomena in the present are the reverberating sensations and feelings inside the body. What is inside becomes an enemy to be avoided to the best of one's ability.

Moreover, when interoceptive information is avoided, other ascending interoceptive signals from the present reality will be regarded as less significant and less valid. The ensuing failure to correctly know bodily states will lead to general homeostatic dysregulation and hence to prolonged interoceptive disturbances with correlated emotional distress—or, in plain English, to prolonged suffering (Khalsa et al. 2018). Another common effect is an insensibility to yourself and your life. This is what happened to Lucía, who was forced to live through chronic verbal and physical abuse over a long period of her childhood.

Lucía was 32 years old and had two children, age 6 and 8 years, and a kind husband. She had been diagnosed with chronic depression and PTSD and had previously tried many different kinds of antidepressants. At the point when we meet her in the dialogue that follows, she has been receiving medication and repetitive transcranial magnetic stimulation (rTMS) treatment. Despite these interventions, the only thing she could think about was suicide. She was unable to work and did very little around the house. She felt numb, out of touch with her family, herself, and life.

Lucía: Clinical Example on Long-Term Effects of Experiential Avoidance of the Body

The eldest of four siblings, Lucía took care of many of the household chores while growing up, and she tried to protect her sisters and brother from abuse by her parents. When Child Protective Services agents came to investigate complaints of child abuse and neglect, she repeatedly told them that everything was fine in order to protect her parents, who were addicted to alcohol. She somehow managed to carry on with her life until 5 years ago, when she became increasingly depressed, and almost continuous thoughts of suicide began to hang over her and her family.

In response to her childhood abuse, Lucía became completely numb to her body's inner states. This numbing resulted in a continuous sense of alienation from herself and from her surroundings, including members of her immediate family. Having lost connection with herself, she had also lost connection with the world. Lucía's habit of disregarding information about the actual state of her body and her feelings also meant that the positive things in her present existence went unrecognized, and she was left with perpetual feelings of meaninglessness and guilt.

It is helpful to think of ascending prediction errors as broadcasting "newsworthy" information—that is, present events that can't be explained by descending predictions based on prior knowledge (see Figure 5–3) give rise to perceptions. The larger the magnitude and the higher the precision weight, the more likely the prediction error is to give rise to perception and learning (i.e., updating beliefs and models). It is thus the relative precision weights of the prediction error and the prior knowledge that decide how much influence each has in what is experienced. However, the brain can also *select* the prediction errors to which it attends or that it ignores, by *assigning* various precisions to ascending bodily signals (Seth and Friston 2016).

Within the framework of interoceptive predictive coding, the neglect of ascending bodily information correlates with assigning it less importance and certainty than the prior model that already exists. Such underestimation of the validity of actual bodily input is framed as affording it less "precision weight"—just as the precision of visual prediction errors is expected to be lower at dusk than in broad daylight.

When someone feels overwhelmed and unable to resolve large prediction errors, either by taking action to change the world to fit the model or by updating beliefs to make the model fit the world, the only response remaining is to decrease the precision weight of the prediction error itself. This, in effect, mutes the signaling system. When this strategy of neglecting bodily signals is applied over time, any ascending bodily information will be underrated (Friston 2020). Models based on prior learning gain unwarranted precision and stability, which makes them yet more resistant to revision based on present experience. This both initiates and sustains a vicious circle of crisis instigation.

Overreliance on Bodily Prior Knowledge

Lucía's interoceptive disturbance—experienced largely as depression, numbing, and disconnection—is based on *underweighting* signals from the body. We return to Lucía later in this chapter to illustrate how the underweighting of bodily information can be tackled through mindfulness of body. First we consider other instances of biased precision weighting, one of which is the problem of assigning too much precision weight to prior knowledge.

When strong beliefs are held that a certain model is correct, regardless of incoming somatic information, the precision of the predictions based on that model is *overweighted*. This creates distinct expectations concerning bodily sensations when one enters certain situations. For example, if one encounters a cue that previously has predicted danger through model-free or model-based learning, this prediction will adjust the observed bodily state to accord with the expected bodily state. In other words, an inner correction will make the bodily sensations match with prior knowledge. A person who has witnessed a shooting, for example, may respond with an oversensitized interoceptive stress response to any type of loud noise (a cue that previously predicted danger), leading to accumulative stress with long-term consequences for physiological and mental health (e.g., Kletter et al. 2021).

Kai, whom we met in Chapter 2 and will meet again in Chapter 7 ("Engagement"), strongly anticipated feeling fearful and anxious when he was around other people. When he was getting ready to board a bus, this prior model generated predictions with high precision weight, which accelerated his breathing and pulse rate. As an aspect of his panic disorder, he also had a prior belief that an elevated heart rate, quickened breathing, and dizziness signified an impending heart attack. Such a belief naturally evokes fear in relation to these changing sensations, and hence a hypervigilant focus upon them, and that fear can quickly escalate into panic.

Behavioral Avoidance of Present Bodily Events

Kai's expectations of fear went hand in hand with his withdrawal from the kinds of pursuits that would cause his heart to beat faster. This behavioral avoidance was a way for him to ensure his incoming physiological sensations match his desired model of calm. When the ascending prediction error is temporarily reduced through behavioral avoidance, producing a temporary experience of relief, such avoidance behavior is negatively reinforced and so becomes the preferred strategy with respect to any potential situation that could possibly provoke disturbing bodily sensations. As we saw in Chapter 2, behavioral avoidance of this kind brings a host of other problems in relating to the world: the rapid loss of functional capacities and the strengthening of dysfunctional prior beliefs about the inner and outer worlds. Voilà—an impending anxiety disorder.

Anxiety disorders are sustained by upregulating bodily responses to match prior fearful models as well as by withdrawing from or avoiding stressful situations that might trigger prediction errors related to the desired model of calm. These ways of changing the body to match the model do feed a sense of agency, but in a problematic way, because these strategies produce only short-term effects. Ultimately, this will lead to a loss of agency and self-efficacy. Kai neither wants to be present to his inner reality nor learn that his model of danger is invalid, so he also misses out on the experience of being present to what is truly there for him in the moment. He has cut himself off from the avenues that lead to mindful doing and being.

Overreliance on Avoiding Unwanted States and Pursuing Desired Ones

An inclination to behavioral or emotional avoidance need not require a past experience of trauma or danger. A fixation on pursuing particular desired states can become a leitmotif of everyday life and will produce unhelpful and unhealthy consequences. If you see a combination of happiness, satisfaction, and calm to be the ideal or even normal state, to be achieved at all times in all settings, you will interpret any deviation from this state as problematic; you will feel a squeak of discrepancy that may be exacerbated by images in advertisements and on social media of other people's seemingly perfect and joyful lives. This discrepancy corresponds to a prediction error between desired and observed internal states, and the prediction error brings a motivation to resolve it through some regulatory response. With repeated exposure to these social messages, we assign ever more precision weight to the desired models, which makes them resistant to change.

Through much of history, people have pursued specific desired—sometimes unachievable—inner states and avoided other experiences. Although strategies that seek to elicit pleasing feelings and avoid negative ones have proven to serve humankind, whose population has steadily increased, evolution doesn't much care about either emotional suffering or lasting happiness. Indeed, if abiding happiness and sustainability are what we want, our evolutionary programming to seek and to avoid has ceased to be adaptive. This notion of evolution gone awry reflects one of the Buddha's central messages: that the root of suffering lies in grasping for and clinging to things that give rise to transient pleasurable states.

Through trying to make ourselves feel better by *doing* something, we can easily get too busy and dysphoric. In moving from one thing to another in the hope of experiencing states of happiness that are usually fleeting and rare, we only cause ourselves more stress and unease. We distract ourselves from any feelings that are unaligned with those we desire, and then we wonder where all the time went. Efforts to control others in order to make ourselves happy impede true intimacy. Avoiding cues associated with distressing previous events limits our range of action. We may seek pleasure using alcohol or drugs, and then we use these same substances to resolve the discrepancy between the way we want to feel and the way we do feel. Substance use can be a fantastic short-term remedy for feelings we don't want. Or we may become physically tense around or push down any hurt, pain, or discomfort that begins to arise. If none of these does the trick, we may turn to extreme risk-taking to distract ourselves from our inner disquiet. Whatever means you use, the pursuit of desired feeling states will lead you to avoid all other feeling states and can thus be understood as a form of experiential avoidance.

Contrary to what we may expect, overreliance on taking action can also result in a sense of powerlessness. Failing to ever fully achieve long-desired bodily states eventually becomes a threat to any genuine sense of agency. In other words, a strong prior belief that we *should be able* to control bodily sensations and feelings will over time become a problem itself because it will inevitably give rise to yet another prediction error. Thus, the sense of falling short becomes a recipe for itself. If our best efforts to regulate the stress of a crisis only seem to exacerbate it, what then are we to do?

Crisis Integration—Mindfulness of Body

Fortunately, taking action is not the only way to reduce the disparity between what is actual and what is believed. We may also adjust our expectations to match the actual (Farb et al. 2015). The distinction between taking action (change) and updating prior beliefs (acceptance) is somewhat analogous to the difference between many psychological and psychiatric interventions and mindfulness-based interventions. Often, a correct diagnosis and appropriate pharmaceuticals offer a necessary platform on which the patient can better open up to their pain and change their unhelpful behavior. However, in contrast to seeking to alter bodily and emotional signals by changing, selecting, controlling, or dampening them by various means, mindfulness involves calm, non-interfering observation of bodily sensations and adjusts expectations through acceptance. It's wise to see these two approaches as complementary.

Let's look at two uncomplicated clinical examples of how mindfulness can contribute to crisis integration.

> August had a difficult upbringing and was diagnosed with a personality disorder as a young adult. One afternoon, when he arrived late for a regular check-up with the nurse, he was distressed to the point of having strong suicidal thoughts. His urge toward self-harm caused him to consider seeking inpatient care in the emergency department, but he knew that his part-

ner, tired of all the drama, wouldn't approve of him ending up in the hospital again. Unable to see any way out, August fell into such a panic that he didn't know what to do with himself. Here we see the surfacing of his crisis instigation process. The nurse could have chosen to engage with August on the level of thought, exploring the pros and cons of the alternatives of either going to the emergency room or going home, but instead she guided August to pay mindful attention to his breath. After attending to his body in this way, August realized he had not eaten all day. After having a sandwich and a glass of milk, he felt calm enough to go home.

This vignette illustrates several things: overlooked homeostatic cues can sometimes lead to confusion and distress to the point of panic; mindfulness neither requires previous experience nor has to be time consuming and can move things forward quickly in unexpected ways; and the body can provide valuable guidance for decision-making.

Like August, Riki had been diagnosed with a personality disorder. She attended an ACT group, and at her third meeting she spoke up to share how she often called her friends when she became so anxious and desperate that she was having suicidal thoughts. This had strained her friendships to the point that she now had only a few friends left. She had also noticed that, even if the phone calls helped temporarily, her sense of inner turmoil often reappeared the same day. On one occasion during the past week, she had tried to refrain from picking up the phone and instead paid attention to her breathing: she witnessed the sensations of her body in a state of full alarm while she followed her value of respecting her friends' time and energy.

"And you know what?" she concluded. "The panic eventually disappeared!"

The other group members were hanging on her every word, both envious and inspired, far more engaged than when the group leader spoke.

This example speaks to the benefits of experiencing ACT in a group context. It also shows that when you don't intervene to try to change distressing bodily sensations, you learn directly that they are transient, having a beginning, middle, and end. What we experience as attending to bodily sensations equates—in terms of predictive coding—to granting greater precision weight to interoceptive prediction errors (Friston 2020). What is important to keep in mind is that this direction of attention *could* make use of a prior belief of danger, in which case the sensations in question will again produce an urge to control or avoid them. Mindful attention, however, will launch from a model one level up in the hierarchy from the belief of danger, and so the belief of danger will become the evidence for a prediction error at the next level up, now pertaining to equanimous meta-awareness. At any point in time and at any level of processing, an individual can have access to numerous models and can hold a belief as to how likely each of these models is to be a true representation of the world (Smith et al. 2021). This turns out to be decisive when one applies mindfulness to gain more insight into bodily and emotional processes and to improve psychological flexibility. In the next part of this chapter, we discuss why that is so. We explore in more depth the clinical implications of the simple but vital skill of mindfulness of body as well as gain some understanding of how it can be understood in terms of predictive coding. Different stages of this kind of work are offered here that, in practice, do not necessarily follow one another in a neat and orderly way. On the whole, these different steps are best seen as steps of an improvised dance. Before entering the dance floor, however, it's useful to master the first move of mindfully attending to a neutral body area.

Mindfulness of Body to Find a Safe Haven

Crisis integration through mindfulness of body preferably begins with identifying neutral areas of the body in which the patient can rest their attention. The emotional neutrality will help to establish the calm, still, witnessing stance that is necessary to stay with, observe, and receive other, more turbulent somatic sensations. With time, these emotionally neutral locations in the body will provide a safe haven wherein the patient can return and rest their attention whenever their suffering becomes too much.

The psychiatrist taught Maurice, for example, to focus on his feet when his emotions threatened to overwhelm him. Marina, meanwhile, found in mindfulness of breath a reprieve from the exhausting and looping thoughts about fear of social rejection due to her HIV diagnosis.

As a rule of thumb, neutral bodily sites are usually located outside the torso, the area of the body where the viscera reside and that is commonly associated with the subjective experiencing of emotions. Attending to the torso as a first step in mindfulness of the body risks the patient quickly slipping into a turmoil of intense and frightening emotions that will immediately trigger avoidance strategies. It's a matter for individual experimentation, but some good places to direct mindful attention include the hands, the feet, or the buttocks if supported by the ground or a chair. Sensations in the spine, or any of the extremities, while making slight movements also provide a good anchor for attention. If sitting still is difficult, the slow movements of tai chi, qi gong, or yoga can support mindfulness. These practices sometimes also bring the discovery of tensions that have been held for so long that they have been totally pushed outside of awareness. Mindful movements will help reveal tensions and wake up ignored body parts. However, such physical exercises can easily be practiced without mindfulness, as a mechanical movement of arms and legs in the air; thus, guidance may be needed to help a patient remain aware of how the body feels from within.

If every part of the body turns out to be too difficult to stay with, one may need to begin with sounds, or anything else that is immediately present, to provide a focus. For some, walking in nature offers a safe resource: you can attend to the sounds of footsteps or birdsong or closely observe an interesting plant. Simplicity is preferable, in order to avoid slipping into thinking and hence failing to be aware and meta-aware of the present moment.

Whenever possible, it is valuable to spend longer periods of time cultivating the ability to rest one's attention in neutral places. After someone has gained proficiency in nurturing tranquility in this way, they may be better prepared to open up attention to bodily areas holding emotional pain. It is also beneficial to learn about self-compassionate ways of relating to oneself, which we address in Chapter 6, "Acceptance and Self-Compassion."

Mindfulness of Body to Reveal What's Hidden

When the time is right, mindfulness of neutral bodily areas provides a means of entry into recognizing and exploring bodily and emotional distress, just as it can later provide somewhere to return to ground yourself. Without that important means of regulating feelings, the experience of acute discomfort may escalate beyond one's ability to stay mindful when starting to open up to difficult history or present loss.

For some people in crisis, mindfulness of any body area, however distant from the torso, will immediately reveal painful emotions. In these cases, the cultivation of mindfulness of body for the sake of experiencing rest will have to go hand in hand with learning more about the emotional pain the crisis brings. For example, Maurice let go of his avoidance strategies for a moment when he slowed down to pay mindful attention to his feet. This enabled him to assign greater precision weight to ascending interoceptive information relative to his prior model of staying "calm"—or, more accurately, staying numb inside. Because he was in the middle of dealing with an enormous loss, sensations of alarm and acute emotions made themselves known immediately. As we see later, Lucía's body also delivered a prompt emotional response when she started to pay attention to it. In a sequence of exchanges with Lucía, we unpack how mindfulness of body can be used to regulate such emotional responses and listen to the information they provide.

It's important to remember that crisis integration requires that the psychiatrist not only nurture a patient's inner resources but also help them secure outer resources and safety. Ongoing abuse and other sources of threat must come to an end. Sources of social support in the form of family, friends, and community or spiritual groups need to be identified and actively recruited to help a patient in crisis. Most importantly, deep trust needs to be established between psychiatrist and patient. People in crisis will take comfort from a sincere, interested listener, especially at times when they are unable to give comfort to themselves. If you're going to explore dangerous territory, you need to know that you are seen and heard and that what you say is taken seriously.

If you are seen with clear, accepting, and loving eyes, your maladaptive response patterns become less a source of shame, do not need to be disguised, and thereby open up to change. It is all about a sharing of reality and obtaining access to supportive and mindful witnessing. If you experience all alone the effects of someone crossing your boundaries, for example, or, even worse, if what has happened to you is dismissed as invalid, there is little to keep you from self-blame or concluding that you deserved what happened (van der Kolk 2015, p. 176). If someone on whom you depend—a parent, teacher, coach, or religious or spiritual teacher—will not validate what you share with them, even a comparably minor transgression of your boundaries can linger within you, causing incredible confusion and suffering. The same goes for losses, accidents, and other stressful events. The long-term adverse effect is to a large extent the result of experiential avoidance, whether this avoidance comes from you or is imposed by others.

Lucía had experienced major abuse throughout her childhood and had received neither care nor validation. In those circumstances, the only available protective mechanism was to put a lid on her inner experiences. As an adult, she has been lucky to build a safe domestic situation in which she can start to investigate what she has kept stored inside and learn to relate to this in a different way. Let's see how mindfulness of body begins to reveal some of her pain.

Lucía—Clinical Dialogue on Mindfulness of Body Bringing Forth Tears

For the past month, Lucía has been taking part in an ACT group for suicidal patients. She has come to all the weekly meetings, but she hasn't taken an active part in the discussion, has made very little eye contact, and has preferred to sit outside the circle. For that reason, she immediately caught the attention of the psychiatrist leading the group when she spoke up at the fifth meeting.

Lucía: I'm not able to do the mindfulness homework.

Psychiatrist: Thank you for telling me that. Would you like to tell me some more about it?

Lucía: I just can't do it. I don't understand any of this.

Psychiatrist: Aha, so that's what's hard—the understanding part?

Lucía: Well, no…yes…I don't know. I just can't do it.

Psychiatrist: Am I right in guessing that you might be interested in trying out mindfulness if you just knew how?

Lucía: Yeah, I guess.

Psychiatrist: (*Waits silently.*)

Lucía: Being present with the breath and sensing the body from within— what *is* that? I just don't get what you mean!

Psychiatrist: That's a really good question. I'm not sure I can explain it very well in words. Maybe instead you could try something with me right now?

Lucía: (*Looks down.*)

Psychiatrist: I'll try to explain it as best I can as we go along.

Lucía: (*Continues looking down.*)

Psychiatrist: In fact, we can do the whole thing together as a group. How does that sound?

Lucía: (*Nods slightly.*)

Psychiatrist: Mindfulness really can be easy, but it can be difficult as well. Let's just see if we can begin somewhere. I suggest we choose a body part at one of our extremities—say, the right big toe. Is that okay? You can look down at your lap if it's easier to concentrate that way. So, can you feel your big toe? You can wiggle it a bit. Notice how the movement feels, the pressure of your shoe under the toe, how the big toe sits beside the next toe. Can I check in with you, Lucía? Is this possible for you to do?

Lucía: Yeah, I can feel my big toe.

Psychiatrist: That's excellent. And now *maybe* you can observe how the *inside* of the toe feels? The toe, sort of from the inside out? Then, when you feel ready, you can leave the big toe—maybe say "thank you" to it and tell it you'll be back later to give it some more attention. That's plenty for now.

Lucía: Was that mindfulness? To feel my toe?

Psychiatrist: Yes, that's what we're after. To feel the toe. Or, to be precise, to be *aware* of the sensations in the toe.

Lucía: "To be aware of the sensations in the toe"?

Psychiatrist: You direct your attention to your toe, as if you were pointing a flashlight at something in the dark. It's there, but you can't see it until you put your flashlight on it. This flashlight is like your attention—shining on your toe. Your attention is right there. (*Points to Lucía's toe.*) But whereas you'd use a flashlight for things outside of your body, you're using your attention to do this on the inside. Okay?

Lucía: Okay. Weird, but okay.

Psychiatrist: You can attend to the place where the toe meets the shoe, for example. Can you notice how that exact spot feels right now? Maybe there's a slight pressure. You can use your attention to zero in on your toe, so you *know* what it is you're sensing. The pressure from the shoe, for example. Are you with me?

Lucía: Sort of.

Psychiatrist: Good! You can experiment with this at home. Would you be willing to have a go at attending to your big toe a few times between now and next week? Only for a few seconds at a time, that's plenty! We'll take it from there next time.

When working with patients with a history of trauma, it is valuable to go slowly. In the best of all worlds, it might well be preferable to work one-on-one with a patient like Lucía over a long period of time. Unfortunately, that is often not an option, depending what mental health resources are locally available. At other times, it may be the patient's choice to decline to work alone with a therapist. That was the case for Lucía. She felt she had come to the end of the rope in trying different interventions but had nevertheless expressed interest—when the opportunity was offered—in joining a group with other patients with suicidality.

At the group meeting the next week, Lucía reported with a confused expression on her face that she had cried for hours the first time she had done the toe exercise by herself. She hadn't dared do the exercise again.

Lucía: What was *that* all about? I mean, all that crying?

Psychiatrist: I'm hearing that you're more curious and puzzled than angry and scared?

Lucía: Sure, I'm not angry, but it was a bit scary. I couldn't stop crying. It just went on and on.

Psychiatrist: Yes, that would certainly feel a bit scary and confusing if it happened to me. Now, I don't know everything about what you've been through, but it is possible there may have been one or two things to cry about in your life. Maybe things you didn't let yourself cry about at the time?

Lucía: Well… (*sigh*)

Psychiatrist: We don't need to go into any of that right now. But I'm curious if any thoughts or images came up while you were focusing on your toe.

Lucía: No, I don't think so, but I only did it for a few seconds before all the crying started.

Psychiatrist: And during the crying? Was anything else going on besides the crying and the scariness of not being able to make it stop?

Lucía: I don't think there was very much. I don't remember everything. I guess I was busy crying my eyes out and trying to get it to stop.

Psychiatrist: And afterward, when eventually it stopped, how did you feel then?

Lucía: Relieved it had finally stopped.

Psychiatrist: Okay, I just wanted to check whether anything else besides the tears had come up that we needed to consider. So about the crying: it seems to me that during those few moments of being aware how your toe felt, your other mechanisms that usually keep you from crying, or feeling things you don't want to feel (*Presses his hands downward in front of his torso.*), actually relaxed for a moment (*Lifts his hands away.*) and so the tears could come out.

Lucía: (*Looks silently at the psychiatrist.*)

Psychiatrist: For children—and adults too—when horrible things happen to them, often the only thing they can do is close down all their reactions, their emotions, and the panic in their body. After a time, it's like having a safe deposit box at the bank: you don't even know it's there and you don't know what's in it until you go to the bank and open it. It can be scary to open it. People often work hard to keep it locked up.

Lucía: Uh-huh.

Psychiatrist: Even thoughts about suicide can help keep that safe deposit box locked up. Frightening as those thoughts may be, they keep us busy and unaware of the *other* frightening and confusing things going on inside us.

Lucía: (*Looks at the psychiatrist in silence and nods*)

Psychiatrist: A safe deposit box like that, within you, may have helped you survive some of the awful things that happened, and I'm super glad you discovered a way through them. The downside is that, as an adult, that very strategy to close down your inner life is sapping so much of your energy.

Lucía: I think I can see what you mean.

Psychiatrist: You know, the fact that you keep coming to this group could mean that you're curious to learn something new. I suspect that you're onto something with the toe exercise. When you feel the time is right to give mindfulness another try, I'll be ready to give you a tool to use when the tears are flooding and you're starting to feel overwhelmed.

Mindfulness of Body to Increase Distress Tolerance and Rediscover the Body

Crucial on the route toward increased distress tolerance is the capacity to witness what is going on, rather than becoming consumed by it or avoiding it. It's not helpful, and can be quite scary, to simply reexperience past events as though they were taking place right now. Even the slightest bit of meta-awareness of emotional experiences in the present moment will be helpful. It's a capacity that often needs to be nurtured through gentle reminders from a listening professional.

In hindsight, it might therefore have been better to help Lucía learn more about how to contact neutral body areas, and remain meta-aware of these, in the group setting before inviting her to try the toe exercise as homework. On her own, just a few seconds of mindfulness of body opened up a few hours of tears. If she, at this point, had already developed a proficiency to reestablish attentional contact with the toe, she could have regained access to meta-awareness. This would have reduced the sense of danger and, instead of having to be so busy trying to stop the tears, Lucía would have felt more able to allow and receive them.

Nevertheless, because Lucía was interested enough to keep attending the group meetings, she had the opportunity to catch up on learning how to return to meta-awareness of a neutral bodily area as a tool to regulate the sense of danger connected to her bodily and emotional experiences. This process has been described as returning to the "islands of safety" (van der Kolk 2015, p. 247).

In dealing with crisis, acute or prolonged, it is best to guide the patient to open up to locked-up distress in a gradual way. Their attention can be carefully directed back and forth between the emotional response within the torso and the sensations in more neutral parts of the body. When one is close to feeling overwhelmed, it is wise to take one's attention back to a more neutral place in which to find rest and equilibrium before once again exploring some charged territory.

Lucía: Clinical Dialogue on Increasing Distress Tolerance by Attending Alternately to Charged and Neutral Bodily Areas

After a few more meetings of her ACT group, Lucía expressed a wish to try again to practice some mindfulness of body. With the psychiatrist's assistance, she established all of her toes and both soles of her feet as her "islands of safety." This was to give her a better sense of the support of the ground under her feet. The rest of the group were asked to support her process by directing their mindful attention to their own feet. As she was being guided through the exercise in being mindful of her toes and the soles of her feet, her breathing became jerky, and her shoulders slumped.

Psychiatrist: How are you doing Lucía? Give me a sense of what's going on right now.
Lucía: It's hard.
Psychiatrist: Yes, it's hard.... Anything else?
Lucía: I don't know. It's just very tight, here. (*Moves her hand to her chest.*) I can't breathe.
Psychiatrist: You're noticing tightness in your chest. It's so tight that you can hardly breathe. Thank you. Let's go back to being aware of your toes and the soles of your feet for a little while. Notice the sensations

of the soles touching the floor, the stillness of your toes, and perhaps some tiny, tingling vibrations inside the toes.
Lucía: Okay. (*Takes a deep breath in and sighs it out.*)

When the past shows up in the present, here in the form of tightness,
what is needed is not to try to work out exactly what event in the past is
causing these sensations but to help the patient tolerate them without being overwhelmed by them (van der Kolk 2015, p. 176). The psychiatrist offers Lucía an alternative to her usual avoidance strategies (e.g., numbness
to bodily sensations or thinking suicidal thoughts) by guiding her attention back to her feet. The sensing of her toes and soles provides both an
entry point from which she can start to receive bodily information *and* a
resting place and anchor for when the discomfort gets too much. Directing one's attention in this way is not an avoidance move; it is a technique
to reestablish meta-awareness and hence regulate the intensity of what is
experienced.

Central to practicing mindfulness of body is the intention to stay with
the physical sensations as much as possible. This means noticing sensations in terms of their sensory properties—"sticky," "sharp," "dense," "spa-
cious," "wobbly," "hard," "soft," "tense"—rather than labeling them in terms
of feelings: "shame," "lonely," "envy," "scared," "sad." In the same vein, it can
be helpful to delay any appraisal, conceptualization, or application of pre-
conceived notions in response to the sensations. In mindfulness of body,
we do not primarily focus on longer narratives about what is coming up.
Premature interpretations can sometimes bring a touch of experiential
avoidance of the sensations, often pertaining to a prior model, and risk
missing the real and full meaning of the bodily information.

There is absolutely nothing wrong with feeling words such as "sad,"
"worried," or "content" in and of themselves. In Chapter 4, the naming of
feelings as they showed up was used as a means to remain meta-aware of
them. There is plenty of science to show that an inability to accurately la-
bel discrete emotions is associated with psychiatric disorders and poorer
physical health. Conversely, adaptive functioning is associated with a
greater ability to know one's emotions (see Smith et al. 2019). However,
the immediate goal of mindfulness of body is to refine the perception of
bodily sensations as they are; the cultivation of this ability will lead in due
course to a more nuanced lexicon of feeling words (e.g., Gibson 2019).

Furthermore, reporting directly on any observed bodily sensations,
especially when they pertain to trauma, helps neutralize the unhealthy
tendency to lapse into a narrative designed to explain why these experiences are present (Segal et al. 2006). It is less important to know why they
are happening than it is to pay witness to them so that they cease to be

seen as threats to be eliminated. Direct observation of bodily sensations also brings validation that what happened was indeed grave. You may then, together with the psychiatrist, explore the specific ways it was grave and into the strategies you have employed thus far to survive.

Well-acquainted with these considerations, the psychiatrist encourages Lucía to stay with bodily sensations at this point.

Lucía: Clinical Dialogue on Staying with Bodily Sensations and Hearing Their Message

> Psychiatrist: Now, slowly, very slowly, move your attention back to your chest, as if to take a little peek at the tightness. Maybe you could even describe it a little. For example, how big is it? (*pause*) How much of your chest does it seem to take up? (*pause*) Is it flat or round? (*pause*) Are there any edges to the area of tightness? (*pause*) Does it border anything else?

By offering examples of how bodily sensations can be described (Gendlin 1982, pp. 43–44), the psychiatrist cues Lucía to remain observant and meta-aware of the sensations. Listening to the body with curious and open-minded attention allows spontaneous new insights to arise; revelations that will counter urges to "do something" that are driven by reactivity to previous learning.

> Lucía: I don't know…. It's very dark.
> Psychiatrist: I see. Do you mean "dark" in the sense that you cannot see anything, or is it that the tightness is dark?
> Lucía: The tightness is very dark and cloggy. (*Bends over and starts to cough.*) They're just too big…my parents…and…I'm just too small. I just can't…protect…myself (*Coughs again.*) or anyone.
> Psychiatrist: They are indeed too big. And there is some coughing going on. Anytime you want to take a little break, you can go back to focusing on your feet again. It's okay to do that anytime you want.
> Lucía: (*Coughing subsides.*) I just feel like I want to cough it all up, you know, the tightness, as if something was stuffed down into me. (*long pause*) You know, I couldn't do anything, couldn't say "no" or fight back. Or if I did, it would get worse. I just couldn't do anything to make them stop. It's as if my "no" was stuffed down.
> Psychiatrist: I guess that's how it feels to be overpowered, right? Having your "no" stuffed down?
> Lucía: Yeah, that's it.
> Psychiatrist: This may sound like a weird idea, but maybe you could thank the tightness in your chest and the cough for

letting you hang out with them and learn something about
them. You can keep your eyes focused on your lap for a little
while. When you're ready, bring yourself back into the room.

After Lucía has experienced and described the bodily sensations, she
is able to gain a bit more insight into what they are related to. The suggestion that she offer some gratitude to her sensations for showing up encourages in her a caring and acknowledging new way of relating to them,
in contrast to her old habit of avoiding and suppressing them.

Mindfulness of body allowed Lucía to practice *leaning in*, to directly
experience the tightness in her chest and the difficulty breathing; *leaning
out*, to reestablish meta-awareness of sensations in her toes and the soles
of her feet; *continuing to lean out*, directing her meta-awareness from her
feet to the tightness in her chest and describing that a bit; and, when she
was ready, *leaning back in*, to directly experience the tightness and the
urge to cough. Simply put, she was "in it" as well as "with it" (Sucitto 2021).
With gentle and interactive guidance, she can, in this alternating way,
gradually build the internal resources to receive and hold all the pain.

Everything that cannot be processed, correctly understood, or integrated at the time of a traumatic event is stored in the body—as van der
Kolk (2015) described in *The Body Keeps the Score*. When Lucía experiences the calming touch of mindfulness of body, she is able to listen to
what the body has to say about the horror, pain, bewilderment, loss, loneliness, and betrayal that she has previously experienced. Gradually she
will begin to trust that she has the capacity, and knows how, to hear the
body's full message. This will not be a comfortable process for her; there
is a reason why the body's voice has been ignored. However, when she receives these bodily responses in meta-awareness, they'll seem less auton-
omous, all-consuming, frightening, and unruly, just as trolls are rendered
harmless by sunlight in Scandinavian folk tales. She will begin to recognize that these unpleasant feelings are the residue of bad things that happened in the past and do not signify ongoing threats in the present. In this
way, the influence of the past on the present is reduced.

Let us ascertain, in terms of predictive coding, how mindfulness can
increase the tolerance of distress and enable the body to be rediscovered.
Directing attention to her feet enables Lucia to establish a tranquil meta-
awareness. This observing position launches from one level up the hierarchy from the prior belief of danger regarding ascending information
from *other* body regions, such as the chest. When meta-awareness is established, the prior *belief* of danger with respect to sensations in the chest
becomes the evidence for the *prediction error* the next level up, the meta-
awareness level. Moreover, a high-precision calm meta-awareness will

downweigh the reliability of the prediction errors based on the evidence of danger, one level down the hierarchy. We discuss more later about how ascending interoceptive information may thereby become ever less likely to be understood in a model of danger and how the range of acceptable sensory input will widen, and thus fewer sensations will demand avoidance techniques, such as suicidal thoughts, to regulate them.

With mindfulness, little by little the body becomes known, witnessed, and reclaimed. This is an iterative process. The more distress that is tolerated, the more the urges, tensions, constrictions, jitters, restlessness, strains, pressures, and aches that have previously been suppressed from awareness will show up to be observed and allowed. Previously avoided bodily distress becomes *exposed* in the imperturbability of the mindfulness state. Lucía's case offers an illustration of "interoceptive exposure."

Mindfulness of Body—Non-systematic Interoceptive Exposure

Since experiential avoidance has a key role in sustaining fear associations (Curreri et al. 2022; Forsyth et al. 2006; Hayes et al. 1996), exposure is a mainstay treatment for many affective disorders, especially anxiety and PTSD, which are commonly seen in the aftermath of crises (American Psychiatric Association 2022; National Institute for Health and Care Excellence 2018). A wealth of randomized controlled trials have established its effectiveness (Hofmann et al. 2012). Important to the application of mindfulness of body and emotion is the observation that an *increased* level of fear during the exposure situation is key to reducing the targeted symptoms in the long run (Craske et al. 2008). In the more recently developed protocols, exposure is no longer geared toward reducing the fear level within the session, but rather toward creating a *new* expectation of safety. A shift of assigning more precision weight to the new model of safety than to the old model of danger can occur on a more automatic, unaware level, as in model-free learning, as well as on a more aware level, as in model-based learning. When the latter type of learning is involved, it is essential that the patient be aware of the anticipated feared outcome of the specific danger in question, tolerate the fear response itself, and recognize the present safe situation (Craske et al. 2008; Curreri et al. 2022). This is why the widely used Unified Protocol—a cognitive-behavioral treatment designed to reduce reliance on experiential avoidance across the full range of anxiety and mood disorders—has been updated to include mindfulness during exposure (Barlow et al. 2017).

One important thing to consider is that, since there are usually a multitude of different exteroceptive stimuli that will trigger anxiety in a single patient, exposure must be applied to manifold situations. If instead targeted on distress related to bodily sensations, interoceptive exposure will generalize to all situations the patient associates with fear (Barlow et al. 2016; Boettcher et al. 2016; Boswell et al. 2019; Paulus et al. 2019; Price et al. 2019). This is one more reason why the ACT model of crisis integration centers on mindfulness of body.

In interoceptive exposure, the tolerance of fear relates to bodily sensations and emotions. Instances in which ascending interoceptive signals meet a prior belief of catastrophic significance are particularly challenging. For Kai, an increased heart rate appertained to an impending physiological or psychological breakdown. For Lucía, bodily sensations were associated with danger and feeling overwhelmed. The exploration of bodily sensations is not a walk in the park when you have learned reasons to be fearful; any bump in the road may strongly herald an emergency.

In conventional interoceptive exposure therapy, specific bodily sensations that have been associated with danger are *systematically* presented to foster a *new* belief: "It is safe and tolerable to have this inner experience; it doesn't lead to fatal outcomes." In a systematic interoceptive exposure session addressing panic disorder, for example, the interoceptive sensations to be evoked will be chosen beforehand and deliberately induced. A patient may be asked to run on a treadmill to induce a racing heartbeat or to breathe through a straw to induce shortness of breath. Attention is then directed to these symptoms to challenge prior catastrophic beliefs concerning them. The new model accommodates the idea that the sensations of, for example, a racing heart are safe and tolerable (Boettcher et al. 2016; Craske et al. 1997; Meuret et al. 2018). Similar methods have been successfully applied to PTSD, social anxiety, eating disorders, and substance use disorders, all of which are commonly seen in long-standing crises (Boswell et al. 2015; Dixon et al. 2015; Khoury et al. 2018; Kletter et al. 2021; Wald and Taylor 2008; Zvolensky et al. 2003).

Mindfulness, in contrast, involves *non-systematic* interoceptive exposure (Brensilver 2015). The invitation is to allow *any* interoceptive signal to appear; anything one might experience when profoundly anxious, depressed, or experiencing PTSD-related symptoms is invited to surface. Whatever the patient is ready to know is allowed to show up so it can be exposed to the equanimous witnessing of mindfulness.

It's important to recognize that attention to bodily symptoms can be both *dysfunctional*—increasing suffering, instigating crisis—and *func-*

tional (Mehling 2016)—reducing suffering, as in crisis integration. Dysfunctional attention to bodily sensations rides on a prior belief of danger, whereas functional mindful attention to what is going on inside comes from the meta-awareness level, one level up the hierarchy from the prior belief of danger. When ascending bodily sensations meet predictions based on a fearful prior model, an avoiding or controlling response is commonly elicited, and the fearful model remains unchallenged and reinforced.

Once high-level equanimous meta-awareness is established, however, the prior belief of danger regarding certain bodily sensations becomes the evidence for a prediction error one level up—the meta-awareness level. For example, when Lucía's shoulders slumped, and she had difficulty breathing, she was guided to reestablish calm meta-awareness through attending to her emotionally neutral "islands of safety" (the toes and soles of her feet). Then her attention was guided to sensations from more emotionally charged areas of the body (the tightness in her chest). This time, the high precision meta-awareness model downweighted the reliability of the prediction errors arising from past evidence of danger. Lucía was then able to stay with the tightness in her chest for a short while and befriend it a little.

In this way, the degree of bodily sensation that can be tolerated, noticed, and processed will gradually increase. Non-systematic interoceptive exposure is thus accomplished and will in time generate a new model of safety regarding signals from all parts of the body. Regular mindfulness practice will then increase the reliability of this model of safety.

In sum, bodily sensations can be witnessed with an anxious kind of attention, making use of a fearful prior belief, that adds to one's suffering and instigates crisis, or they can be witnessed with a mindful kind of attention that facilitates non-systematic interoceptive exposure and crisis integration. These findings are very important in clinical care in general and in dealing with crisis in particular.

In mindfulness you notice also the *habitual* tendencies to avoid or approach the interoceptive sensations—not only the tendencies learned through your own life experience but also those derived through evolution. Overreliance on "doing something," as described earlier, is rooted in evolutionary-shaped inclinations to avoid or crave certain conditions in order to achieve desirable internal states. The ability to simply notice these inclinations, instead of always acting on them, and then to bring your attention back to the interoceptive sensations is crucial to cultivating psychological flexibility. People sometimes find it difficult to stay observant of the unfolding of interoceptive sensations without moving into approach or avoidance strategies. However, mindfulness of body *slows down* the sequence and thereby expands the opportunities to make appropriate choices.

What seems at first to be enduring and fixed prior knowledge relating to interoceptive cues, shaped through evolution or one's previous experience, can be updated and broadened through moment-to-moment awareness of bodily sensations and of prior knowledge related to them. It is actually simpler than it first seems, if we just remember to gently attend to somatic sensations, the sense of being and having a body—or if, when guiding others toward crisis integration, we remember to bring back an interoceptive focus whenever things are stuck or move too quickly into reactivity.

Mindful Being and Mindful Doing

One communication teacher leading groups of men who'd been convicted of physical abuse asked them to name their present feelings at the end of each meeting, with the condition they not use the words "good" or "bad." They were asked instead to expand their vocabulary to include other words such as "grateful," "relieved," "fascinated," "irritable," "indifferent," or "frustrated" (J. Morrison, personal communication, April 2021). A wealth of studies has shown that a more nuanced and precise knowing of feeling states correlates with better mental health (summarized in Smith et al. 2019) and improves our capacity to take appropriate actions (Lane and Schwartz 1987). Mindfulness of body achieves all this through an intentional and curious examining of bodily information, which in turn refines our perception of corresponding feeling states.

Through mindfulness of body, we can become more confident that the pain will not destroy us, and thus we may feel less intimidated by our inner life. As aspects of our past are allowed to arise into awareness, we learn to accept all that has been stored in our body. As Lucía's dialogue demonstrates, calm witnessing of bodily and emotional distress has the effect down the line of changing the very sensations themselves. Now, if Lucía had set out to be mindful of her body with the *goal* of causing her distressing sensations to change for the better, she would have been deploying another avoidance strategy. She would have been seeking to avoid negative feelings and reach for positive ones, contrary to the way that mindfulness and acceptance actually work.

The phenomenon of wanting less or more of an experience is not an aberration but builds on an inherent inner bias, as described in Chapter 2. As mentioned in Chapter 4, the third dimension of mindfulness addresses exactly this bias: we become increasingly meta-aware of any desire for or aversion to whatever we're experiencing in the present moment. Chapter 6 unpacks more about how our capacity to accept can be enlarged.

When we are freed from interpreting all that is going on in the present with reference to our past, we can fully enter into life in the here and now.

This in turn increases the accuracy with which we apprehend present feelings, needs, and values, which is essential for our sense of engagement, vitality, and purpose, as we see in Chapter 7.

In this chapter, we explored how mindfulness of body reveals *prior knowledge* based on evolutionary-based, model-free, and model-based learning, as well as one's responses to *present events*, and how this process contributes to psychological flexibility in crisis integration. The Buddha said that "within this fathom-long body" is found all the teachings. Having explored the mind solely by means of introspection, William James developed a theory of emotions that, he claimed, "makes us realize more deeply than ever how much of our mental life is knit up on our corporal frame" (James 1890, p. 467). The term *mindfulness of body* is a translation of the Pali *kayagata-sati*, which the Buddha used in introducing this practice. An alternative translation is "mindfulness immersed in the body" (Thanissaro 1997). The Buddha was pointing out that, in the course of time, one's mindful attention should include all of the body. Although mindfulness of body usually starts with attending to one single object, such as the breath or, as in Luciá's case, the big toe, it eventually encompasses the whole body. In this endeavor, it is helpful to perceive one's body as fairly safe to reside within.

By increasing our familiarity with the inner world of the body, we can let go of being on our guard lest we encounter something surprising, unknown, and threatening. A momentary body scan becomes less like entering a minefield and more like drifting in a flower-filled pasture. Although the inner world may include ravines, jungles, and swamps, and the weather there is sometimes stormy, we gradually learn to trust that the body is a safe enough place to enter and explore. A loving relationship with one's body, lost through painful experiences or through habit, can be reestablished through relatively simple mindfulness practice. It is a path worth taking. The body becomes a place of sanctuary when we don't know what else to do with all the confusion and distress of a crisis. It also enables us to shift focus from running away from what is happening inside to recognizing and incrementally embracing it. This frees us from the prison of avoidance, control, and elimination strategies so that our actions may become motivated by authentic values and needs.

Truly, the more comfortable we feel within our own skin, the more we become at home in the world. Awareness of body facilitates positive experiences that impart a growing sense of vitality. Little sparks of joy may be ignited by acts of kindness or by the sensory delights of food, fragrance, music, art, and nature. The body can in these ways become a trustworthy source of respite, learning, guidance, and gladness.

When we choose to receive and stay with what is going on within, we will let the sensations be as they are in this moment. In the ACT model of crisis integration, such presence is the foundation of "mindful being" and acceptance. Through mindfulness, we also learn what is important to us in the short and long term, and thus our inner experiences function as messengers that can guide our actions. Hence the "mindful doing," or engagement, component of the ACT approach, which helps restore our sense of agency—the self-efficacy that crisis science has found so beneficial to recovery from unexpected catastrophic events (Southwick et al. 2011).

Acceptance and engagement are interwoven with mindfulness of body. As we become more aware of our body's present state, we become better able to take care of it—that is, of ourselves. In knowing how to accept and take care of our inner world, we become more adept at engaging with and caring for our outer world and the people who matter to us.

References

American Psychiatric Association: Diagnostic and Statistical Manual of Mental Disorders, 5th Edition, Text Revision. Washington, DC, American Psychiatric Association, 2022

Armstrong K: How we understand our body's inner sensations. September 25, 2019. Available at: https://www.psychologicalscience.org/observer/interoception-how-we-understand-our-bodys-inner-sensations. Accessed May 28, 2021.

Barrett LF, Simmons WK: Interoceptive predictions in the brain. Nat Rev Neurosci 16(7):419–429, 2015 26016744

Bauernfeind AL, de Sousa AA, Avasthi T, et al: A volumetric comparison of the insular cortex and its subregions in primates. J Hum Evol 64(4):263–279, 2013 23466178

Barlow DH, Allen LB, Choate ML: Toward a unified treatment for emotional disorders—republished article. Behav Ther 47(6):838–853, 2016 27993336

Barlow DH, Sauer-Zavala S, Ellard KK, et al: Unified Protocol for Transdiagnostic Treatment of Emotional Disorders: Therapist Guide. Oxford, UK, Oxford University Press, 2017

Bayes TR: An essay towards solving a problem in the doctrine of chances. Philos Trans R Soc Lond 53:370–418, 1763

Boettcher H, Brake CA, Barlow DH: Origins and outlook of interoceptive exposure. J Behav Ther Exp Psychiatry 53:41–51, 2016 26596849

Boswell JF, Anderson LM, Anderson DA: Integration of interoceptive exposure in eating disorder treatment. Clin Psychol Sci Pract 22(2):194–210, 2015

Boswell JF, Anderson LM, Oswald JM, et al: A preliminary naturalistic clinical case series study of the feasibility and impact of interoceptive exposure for eating disorders. Behav Res Ther 117:54–64, 2019 30797537

Brensilver M: Psychotherapy and Dharma. Dharmaseed (podcast), April 6, 2015. Available at: https://www.dharmaseed.org/talks/26810. Accessed October 19, 2022.

Cannon WB: The Wisdom of the Body. New York, WW Norton, 1932

Carlsson K, Petersson KM, Lundqvist D, et al: Fear and the amygdala: manipulation of awareness generates differential cerebral responses to phobic and fear-relevant (but nonfeared) stimuli. Emotion 4(4):340–353, 2004 15571433

Clark JE, Watson S, Friston KJ: What is mood? A computational perspective. Psychol Med 48:2277-84, 2018

Craig AD: How do you feel? Interoception: the sense of the physiological condition of the body. Nat Rev Neurosci 3(8):655–666, 2002 12154366

Craig AD: Interoception: the sense of the physiological condition of the body. Curr Opin Neurobiol 13(4):500–505, 2003 12965300

Craig AD: How do you feel—now? The anterior insula and human awareness. Nat Rev Neurosci 10:59-70, 2009

Craig AD: How Do You Feel? An Interoceptive Moment with Your Neurobiological Self. Princeton, NJ, Princeton University Press, 2014

Craske MG, Rowe M, Lewin M, et al: Interoceptive exposure versus breathing retraining within cognitive-behavioural therapy for panic disorder with agoraphobia. Br J Clin Psychol 36(1):85–99, 1997 9051281

Craske MG, Kircanski K, Zelikowsky M, et al: Optimizing inhibitory learning during exposure therapy. Behav Res Ther 46(1):5–27, 2008 18005936

Critchley HD, Garfinkel SN: Interoception and emotion. Curr Opin Psychol 17:7-14, 2017

Critchley HD, Harrison NA: Visceral influences on brain and behavior. Neuron 77(4):624–638, 2013 23439117

Curreri AJ, Farchione TJ, Sauer-Zavala S, et al: Mindful emotion awareness facilitates engagement with exposure therapy: an idiographic exploration using single case experimental design. Behav Modif 46(1):36–62, 2022 32752883

Damasio AR: Descartes' Error: Emotion, Reason, and the Human Brain. New York, GP Putnam, 1994

Dixon LJ, Kemp JJ, Farrell NR, et al: Interoceptive exposure exercises for social anxiety. J Anxiety Disord 33:25–34, 2015 25988536

Dolan RJ: Emotion, cognition, and behavior. Science 298(5596):1191–1194, 2002 12424363

English E: Into the Flow: A Gentle Guide to Mindfulness Meditation. Oxford, UK, Mud Pie Books, 2023

Farb N, Segal ZV, Mayberg H, et al: Attending to the present: mindfulness meditation reveals distinct neural modes of self-reference. Soc Cogn Affect Neurosci 2(4):313–322, 2007 18985137

Farb N, Segal ZV, Anderson AK: Mindfulness meditation training alters cortical representations of interoceptive attention. Soc Cogn Affect Neurosci 8(1):15–26, 2013 22689216

Farb N, Daubenmier J, Price CJ, et al: Interoception, contemplative practice, and health. Front Psychol 6:763, 2015 26106345

Fletcher PC, Frith CD: Perceiving is believing: a Bayesian approach to explaining the positive symptoms of schizophrenia. Nat Rev Neurosci 10(1):48–58, 2009 19050712

Flynn FG: Anatomy of the insula functional and clinical correlates. Aphasiology 13:55–78, 1999

Forsyth JP, Eifert GH, Barrios V: Fear conditioning in an emotion regulation context: a fresh perspective on the origins of anxiety disorders, in Fear and Learning: From Basic Processes to Clinical Implications. Edited by Craske MG, Hermans D, Vansteenwegen D. Washington, DC, American Psychological Association, 2006, pp 133–153

Friston KJ: Bayesian dysconnections. Am J Psychiatry 177(12):1110–1112, 2020 33256441

Friston KJ, Daunizeau J, Kilner J, et al: Action and behavior: a free-energy formulation. Biol Cybern 102(3):227–260, 2010 20148260

Frith CD: Making Up the Mind: How the Brain Creates Our Mental World. Oxford, UK, Blackwell, 2007

Frith CD: The neural basis of consciousness. Psychol Med 51(4):550–562, 2021 31481140

Gendlin ET: Focusing, 2nd Edition. New York, Bantam Books, 1982

Gibson J: Mindfulness, interoception, and the body: a contemporary perspective. Front Psychol 10:2012, 2019 31572256

Gizowski C, Bourque CW: The neural basis of homeostatic and anticipatory thirst. Nat Rev Nephrol 14(1):11–25, 2018 29129925

Gu X, Hof PR, Friston KJ, et al: Anterior insular cortex and emotional awareness. J Comp Neurol 521(15):3371–3388, 2013 23749500

Hayes SC, Wilson KG, Gifford EV, et al: Experimental avoidance and behavioral disorders: a functional dimensional approach to diagnosis and treatment. J Consult Clin Psychol 64:1152-68, 1996

Hofmann SG, Asnaani A, Vonk IJ, et al: The efficacy of cognitive behavioral therapy: a review of meta-analyses. Cognit Ther Res 36(5):427–440, 2012 23459093

James W: The Principles of Psychology. New York, Henry Holt, 1890, pp 442–485

Joyce J: A painful case, in Dubliners. London, Grant Richards, 1914

Khalsa SS, Adolphs R, Cameron OG, et al: Interoception and mental health: a roadmap. Biol Psychiatry Cogn Neurosci Neuroimaging 3(6):501–513, 2018 29884281

Khoury NM, Lutz J, Schuman-Olivier Z: Interoception in psychiatric disorders: a review of randomized, controlled trials with interoception-based interventions. Harv Rev Psychiatry 26(5):250–263, 2018 30188337

Kletter H, Matlow R, Tanovic S, et al: Cue-centered therapy for youth experiencing posttraumatic symptoms. Curr Treat Options Psychiatry 8(3):125–140, 2021 33898161

Lane RD, Schwartz GE: Levels of emotional awareness: a cognitive-developmental theory and its application to psychopathology. Am J Psychiatry 144(2):133–143, 1987 3812780

Lane RD, Weihs KL, Herring A, et al: Affective agnosia: expansion of the alexithymia construct and a new opportunity to integrate and extend Freud's legacy. Neurosci Biobehav Rev 55:594–611, 2015 26054794

Löffler A, Foell J, Bekrater-Bodmann R: Interoception and its interaction with self, other, and emotion processing: implications for the understanding of psychosocial deficits in borderline personality disorder. Curr Psychiatry Rep 20(4):28, 2018 29594580

McEwen BS, Stellar E: Stress and the individual: mechanisms leading to disease. Arch Intern Med 153(18):2093–2101, 1993 8379800

Mehling W: Differentiating attention styles and regulatory aspects of self-reported interoceptive sensibility. Philos Trans R Soc Lond B Biol Sci 371(1708):371, 2016 28080970

Meuret AE, Ritz T, Wilhelm FH, et al: Hypoventilation therapy alleviates panic by repeated induction of dyspnea. Biol Psychiatry Cogn Neurosci Neuroimaging 3(6):539–545, 2018 29573981

National Institute for Health and Care Excellence (NICE): Post-traumatic stress disorder (NG116). 2018. Available at: https://www.nice.org.uk/guidance/ng116. Accessed February 21, 2021.

Öhman A, Soares JJF: "Unconscious anxiety": phobic responses to masked stimuli. J Abnorm Psychol 103(2):231–240, 1994 8040492

Öhman A, Carlsson K, Lundqvist D, et al: On the unconscious subcortical origin of human fear. Physiol Behav 92(1–2):180–185, 2007 17599366

Palmer CJ, Seth AK, Hohwy J: The felt presence of other minds: predictive processing, counterfactual predictions, and mentalising in autism. Conscious Cogn 36:376–389, 2015 25934216

Paulus MP, Stein MB: Interoception in anxiety and depression. Brain Struct Funct 214(5–6):451–463, 2010 20490545

Paulus MP, Feinstein JS, Khalsa SS: An active inference approach to interoceptive psychopathology. Annu Rev Clin Psychol 15:97–122, 2019 31067416

Pavlov L: Conditioned Reflexes. Oxford, UK, Oxford University Press, 1927

Price CJ, Thompson EA, Crowell SE, et al: Immediate effects of interoceptive awareness training through Mindful Awareness in Body-oriented Therapy (MABT) for women in substance use disorder treatment. Subst Abus 40(1):102–115, 2019 29949455

Segal ZV, Kennedy S, Gemar M, et al: Cognitive reactivity to sad mood provocation and the prediction of depressive relapse. Arch Gen Psychiatry 63(7):749–755, 2006 16818864

Seth AK: Interoceptive inference, emotion, and the embodied self. Trends Cogn Sci 17:565–73, 2013

Seth AK: Consciousness: the last 50 years (and the next). Brain Neurosci Adv 2:2398212818816019, 2018 32166164

Seth AK, Friston KJ: Active interoceptive inference and the emotional brain. Philos Trans R Soc Lond B Biol Sci 371(1708):371, 2016 28080966

Sherrington CS: The Integrative Action of the Nervous System. New Haven, CT, Yale University Press, 1906

Singer T, Seymour B, O'Doherty J, et al: Empathy for pain involves the affective but not sensory components of pain. Science 303(5661):1157–1162, 2004 14976305

Singer T, Critchley HD, Preuschoff K: A common role of insula in feelings, empathy and uncertainty. Trends Cogn Sci 13(8):334–340, 2009 19643659

Smith R, Killgore WDS, Lane RD: The structure of emotional experience and its relation to trait emotional awareness: a theoretical review. Emotion 18(5):670–692, 2018 29172623

Smith R, Parr T, Friston KJ: Simulating emotions: an active inference model of emotional state inference and emotion concept learning. Front Psychol 10:2844, 2019 31920873

Smith R, Kuplicki R, Feinstein J, et al: A Bayesian computational model reveals a failure to adapt interoceptive precision estimates across depression, anxiety, eating, and substance use disorders. PLOS Comput Biol 16(12):e1008484, 2020 33315893

Smith R, Badcock P, Friston KJ: Recent advances in the application of predictive coding and active inference models within clinical neuroscience. Psychiatry Clin Neurosci 75(1):3–13, 2021 32860285

Southwick SM, Litz BT, Charney D, et al: Resilience and Mental Health: Challenges Across the Lifespan. Cambridge, UK, Cambridge University Press, 2011

Sterling P: Homeostasis vs allostasis: implications for brain function and mental disorders. JAMA Psychiatry 71(10):1192–1193, 2014 25103620

Sucitto A: How to not go crazy. Dharmaseed (podcast), April 21, 2021. Available at: https://www.dharmaseed.org/teacher/9/talk/64839. Accessed October 19, 2022.

Tang YY, Holzel BK, Posner MI: The neuroscience of mindfulness meditation. Nat Rev Neurosci 16:213-25, 2015

Thanissaro B: Kayagata-Sati Sutta: mindfulness immersed in the body. 1997. Available at: https://www.accesstoinsight.org/tipitaka/mn/mn.119.than.html. Accessed May 24, 2021.

van der Kolk B: The Body Keeps the Score: Brain, Mind, and Body in the Healing of Trauma. London, Penguin Books, 2015

von Helmholtz H: Concerning the Perceptions in General: Treatise on Physiological Optics (1866). New York, Dover, 1962

Wald J, Taylor S: Responses to interoceptive exposure in people with posttraumatic stress disorder (PTSD): a preliminary analysis of induced anxiety reactions and trauma memories and their relationship to anxiety sensitivity and PTSD symptom severity. Cogn Behav Ther 37(2):90–100, 2008 18470740

Yoris A, García AM, Traiber L, et al: The inner world of overactive monitoring: neural markers of interoception in obsessive-compulsive disorder. Psychol Med 47(11):1957–1970, 2017 28374658

Zvolensky MJ, Lejuez CW, Kahler CW, et al: Integrating an interoceptive exposure-based smoking cessation program into the cognitive-behavioral treatment of panic disorder: theoretical relevance and case demonstration. Cogn Behav Pract 10(4):347–357, 2003

6

Acceptance and Self-Compassion

We need to let go, to rest, to just be. We need to accept what is, not just mentally, but with the whole of our being, intimately.

—Tara Brach

Crisis Integration With Acceptance

When they reach out for help in a crisis, most patients are seeking help with managing the magnitude of their heartbreak. They may well interpret their continued suffering as an indication that whatever means they've been using to control their pain is inadequate, and the psychiatrist is thus often asked to provide better ways for curtailing their anguish. In the ACT model of crisis, such efforts to *avoid* emotional pain are understood to be the problem rather than the solution.

Instead of trying to change the pain, we help patients develop new ways of *relating* to it—namely, to lean into the pain, to experience it directly (see Figure 4–1, Level 2) while accepting, knowing, and being with it in meta-awareness (see Figure 4–1, Level 3). It then becomes possible to engage with and act on one's values because distressing inner experiences no longer function as barriers to committed action.

The emphasis on promoting acceptance in the ACT model of crisis originates in the recognition that avoidance is the signature of much of our daily activity, to the extent that it largely goes unnoticed. Although acceptance may sound as easy as saying "A-B-C," it is, in fact, a lifelong endeavor to recognize and make peace with all of the avoidance strategies we habitually use in daily life. It wouldn't be farfetched to claim that just about everything we do—both internally and externally—that impedes awareness of our present-moment experience and impedes us from engaging with our values can be understood in terms of experiential avoidance. Acceptance and mindfulness help us to notice fine-spun nuances of avoidance, such as incessantly trying to figure things out, as Marina in Chapter 4 ("A Field Guide to Mindfulness") did whenever she felt afraid and vulnerable. It is crucial to help patients wake up to these ingeniously disguised, personally tailored avoidance strategies or they will otherwise continue to operate behind the scenes, only to take the stage in times of stress.

We use the word *instigation* here in a sense that acknowledges that crisis is not instigated just once and then carried on automatically afterward but involves an ongoing process of re-instigation. When an avoidance strategy is applied to a condition of emotional distress, the crisis is instigated anew. The good news is that, conversely, every time some facet of distress is accepted, crisis *integration* will be under way. Very often, the development of a capacity for meta-awareness and openness to distressing inner experiences is all that's needed for emotional discomfort to lose its power over the patient's behavior. Little by little, the pain of the present moment can be experienced and known. Acceptance thereby incrementally brings about a paradigm shift. However, sometimes meta-awareness and openness bring one into contact with a major barrier to acceptance: a rigid identification with harshly negative beliefs about oneself, or what we may call a "criticized self."

The Self as a Barrier to Acceptance

Identification with and clinging to an inner experience are as much a hindrance to psychological flexibility as avoidance. Attachment and avoidance are two sides of the same coin. One of the nuances of practicing acceptance is learning to let go of attachment to inner experiences. Acceptance often breaks down when a person identifies some aspect of their sense of self that they don't like. A sense of self that is loved is more readily held lightly in acceptance, whereas a sense of self of which one is critical is very sticky. This is not to conflate love with high self-esteem, or indeed with an inflated sense of self, in which again there is a rigid identification with the self. The fact remains that, as long as one firmly identifies with a self, whether criticized or magnified, it is difficult to access the larger perspective conducive to crisis integration. As we shall see, attachment to self-concepts, particularly ones that are harsh and self-rejecting, plays a central role in the origin, development, and maintenance of a psychiatric crisis.

Many of our patients live in close proximity to the metronome of harsh internal criticism. When acceptance is squeezed out by punitive and self-critical evaluations of who you are and who you will become in the future, aversion becomes amplified. This additional negative affect prompts even more experiential avoidance, eventually reducing psychological flexibility to near zero. A self that is seen as flawed and inadequate is highly deleterious to our mental health because it imposes a high level of self-instructional control (see Chapter 2, "The ACT Model of Crisis Instigation"). It tells you that you deserve to expect the worst and sometimes even tells you to behave accordingly. The negative consequences of negative beliefs about the self then roll in relentlessly, exacerbating the crisis.

If the practice of acceptance is neither available nor sufficient to help you relinquish your identification with a criticized self, then what other options do you have? Well, there is something else you can do besides simply noticing the negative judgments about the self and mindfully accepting them without struggle: you can embrace the pain produced by the self-criticism and, at the same time, bathe yourself in kindness and affection. This dual response is part of the practice of self-compassion. In this chapter, we explore the concepts of self and self-criticism, as well as how self-compassion can be applied in the service of unconditional acceptance—and how acceptance and mindfulness bolster self-compassion.

The Self: A Perception Among Other Perceptions

In the absence of meta-awareness, we are "fused" with experience, and we identify with a sense of self. The Buddha noted that such an attachment to a sense of self is a major cause of suffering. When we practice mindfulness, we witness whatever arises for what it is, including our sense of "I" as distinct from the world around us. We neither agree with and cling to the perception of self nor oppose, criticize, and struggle with it; we just accept it as a perception among other perceptions. For anyone strongly identified with the perception of self, this may at first sound radical. The experience of identifying with a self is so familiar, so unified, so continuous that it is difficult even to question it. Let us therefore expand a little on the subject of "self."

In his "Copernican revolution," Immanuel Kant introduced "the subject" as an active originator of experience rather than a passive recipient of perceptions. Kant said that we do not know reality as it is, "das Ding an sich" (the thing in itself); our knowledge about the world is our interpretation of it, "das Ding für mich" (the thing for me) (Kant 1781/1996). Just as Copernicus moved the Earth out of, and the sun into, the center of the universe, Kant moved the "truth" out of, and the subject into, the center of our experience of reality. Kant was on the dot: we can never know how things are, we can only know how things seem to be—as our neural system enables us to experience them. Kant's proposition is aligned with the predictive coding theory described in Chapter 5 ("Mindfulness of Body and Feeling")—except that predictive coding also deconstructs the sense of an existing, true *mich*.

The experience of *mich* or "me" is commonly taken for granted as being true; the self as an enduring entity, something unique that receives information about the world, contemplates alternative actions, and decides what to do next. This is how it seems, but the reality understood by neuroscience is very different. The theory of predictive coding reveals the "self," too, to be a perception (Seth 2021)—and not Kant's "that which does the perceiving." This perception of a "me" emerges from the brain's generating and deploying models of a self, analogous to its use of models for all other types of perceptions.

In Chapter 5, we examined how perception—experiences of the inner and outer worlds—involves two counterflowing streams of signals in the nervous system. One stream conveys predictions about the causes of sensory inputs. The predictions are met with a stream of prediction errors that signal the difference between what the brain gets and what it expects. The neural system continually calibrates its models based on these prediction errors in order to come as close as possible to detecting a useful "truth" of the present moment. Perception thus comes as much, if not more, from predictions based on previous models as from presently incoming information (Seth 2021). Every experience is a construction, an interpretation. We may be willing to agree with this statement insofar as it refers to the perception of the exterior (exteroception) and the body's interior (interoception), but how about the perception of the self?

On a fundamental level, an experience of selfhood emerges because of the body. To know what is part of one's body and what is not is a basic skill that maximizes one's chances of remaining alive. The brain uses exteroceptive organs, such as the eyes, to know that the trunk, the limbs, and other body parts are all attached to each other as part of one singular organism, which adds up to the sense of having a body. Through interoception, the brain "knows" the body from within, which produces the sense of being a body. The body thus plays a key role in structuring one kind of experience of self. But what about other experiences of selfhood?

In ACT, self-related experiences are grouped into three categories, in descending order of their ubiquity in everyday life:

1. *Self-as-content* is the experience of being a continuous self over time, a narrative self that depends on autobiographical memory and the unlimited relational abilities of language and cognition. This experience of a "me" is also shaped by how I perceive others' perception of me while we're interacting. Trouble awaits when identification with self-as-content is framed as judgments of what I *am*—generally some version of good or bad. The Dalai Lama described the "conceptual self" as the clouds that obscure the blue sky of clarity and compassion (The Dalai Lama 2009). The fundamental issues we face in crisis instigation and crisis integration most often originate in difficulties arising from overidentification with the conceptual self.

2. *Self-as-process* pertains to the ongoing and ever-changing inner experiences that show up in awareness if we pay attention: somatic sensations, feelings, thoughts, memories, images, urges, and so on. Self-as-process also includes the ongoing sense of intention and agency, the sense of the self as a cause of things happening in the world. This form of self-experience can be helpful in clinical work—for example, when the psychiatrist asks the patient to perform a slow body scan to identify any areas in which a particular sensation or emotion is manifesting itself. The patient is being asked to be an "observer" of the ongoing appearance of inner experience. This type of "selfing" is generally beneficial because it redirects attention out of the symbolic world of the conceptual self and into the world of immediate perception.

3. *Self-as-context* refers to the perspective of "I," or the world as seen through my eyes and my eyes alone. It can also be used to change perspectives on what "I" means, including ultimately the elimination of "I" as distinct from the rest of humanity. "I" could take on the meaning of a wise, ageless part of the universe or the meaning of having empathy for the suffering of all beings and an endless desire to help alleviate that suffering. These highly expansive self-perspectives are a key focus of skill development in ACT.

All these different experiences of self, like any other experience, build not only on information about the present but also on predictions based on prior knowledge. As Anil Seth (2021) put it, in homage to Descartes, "I predict myself, therefore I am." With practice in mindfulness, you move out of identifying with any of these versions of self, particularly self-as-content. This accords with neuroscience; your brain does not actually contain a homunculus— a miniature self—that experiences and perceives the inner and outer worlds. Our experiences of "selves" are perceptions among other perceptions. However, our social training in selfing teaches us to adopt a literal interpretation of self-as-content: one with a specific history leading to fixed and unchangeable qualities and destined for a specific set of outcomes in the future.

Self-Criticism Exacerbates Crises

Human beings continually try to make sense of what has happened and is happening to them. An ongoing sense of coherence helps us predict the immediate, intermediate, and distant futures. Language provides a convenient vehicle for developing a coherent self-narrative (self-as-content), which can be accessed privately or shared with others. This verbally constructed self-as-content extends into compounded stories about the self that allow us to share our experiences and create social bonds in the process. The dark side of this dynamic is that self-stories can, and do, take on other powerful social functions, such as criticism, rejection, abandonment, and ostracism—in which case they don't produce social bonding but instead produce social isolation and marginalization.

Although there are many kinds of self-critical stories, there are two overarching themes. One emphasizes personal flaws in a self-rejecting or self-hating story. It requires the person to remove perceived flaws in order to avoid ongoing punishment from the world. It typically establishes an impossible rule that "If you want to be happy, complete, and socially accepted, you must first get rid of this defect. If you can't do that, you will be alone, alienated, unloved, and uncared for." The second self-critical theme emphasizes the need to avoid making mistakes and to improve skills or personal attributes that you currently lack (e.g., confidence, competence, strength, kindliness, responsiveness, good looks, social graces) in order to garner approval, inclusion, and safety. Failure to measure up to this self-improvement standard is equivalent to losing the love, care, and affection of others. This story puts tremendous pressure on the individual to over-perform. They work tirelessly to do things for people who matter to them, and when this story gets entangled in all areas of life—work, love, family, and friends—it can quickly lead to burnout, depression, and disability.

Both these forms of self-critical story are difficult to bear, but the self-improvement type is slightly easier because it usually doesn't come with an active resistance to compassion from self and others (Castilho et al. 2017; Gilbert et al. 2011). There is substantial evidence that self-criticism is not only a transdiagnostic symptom but also an important vulnerability factor in the development of depression, anxiety disorders, personality disorders, psychotic symptoms, interpersonal difficulties, self-harm, and suicide risk (Werner et al. 2019).

Marina's case offers a straightforward illustration of how self-critical stories exacerbate crisis instigation. By rebuking and rejecting herself, she added further emotional pain to the pain she was already experiencing for other reasons. Negative self-judgment demanded her attention at the exact moments when she needed to address the demands of the crisis situation. When she was diagnosed with HIV, she experienced deep anguish. If she had been familiar with processes for integrating such a major challenge, she could have attended to and accepted her despair and mourned her loss of health in a helpful way. She could have been angry at the man who had infected her for not being more careful and caring. She could have been upset with herself for not taking better care of herself. Eventually she could have accepted her anger, and maybe she could have forgiven both her sex partner and herself. With the aid of modern medications, she would in due course have been able to live her life fully again. Instead, Marina responded to this sudden negative turn in her life through the lens of a self-rejecting story. This added several new elements to Marina's crisis instigation process:

1. Others' and her own negative judgments of her as a person who'd been infected with HIV (e.g., "I am sullied")
2. The emotional pain of identifying with the judgments about her and the concomitant fears of rejection, exclusion, and social isolation
3. Avoidance of the emotional pain and fear arising from her identification with the negative judgments—most prominently, her incessant thoughts, including suicidal ones

If we were to put a magnifying glass to what was happening in Marina's self-judgments, we would see that one part of her was saying that she was sullied (her verbally constructed self-story) and another part was identifying with the judgment that she was sullied (her overidentification with her self-story).

In this case, relating to what was going on inside with pure acceptance and mindfulness—that is, experiencing, receiving, and witnessing the inner experience—could make her feel confused about what exactly she was supposed to be accepting. For example, in the dialogue in Chapter 4, Marina asked, "If I have the thought that my HIV means I'm sullied, do I have to welcome that as well?" The answer was "yes" *if* she could perceive it as just a thought and not as a truth about herself. Marina was making good progress in taking a meta-aware perspective of her self-deprecating thoughts and emotions. At home, however, as we see later, she came in and out of the ability to let go of her identification with a criticized self. There are certainly many different ways of letting go of identification with a negative self-view. We focus here on two conceptualizations of how to do so. One develops through mindfulness and acceptance, and the other develops through the cultivation of self-compassion. We should keep in mind, however, that although mindfulness, acceptance, and self-compassion each have their own distinct qualities, they unmistakably include aspects of each other because they are all interconnected.

Crisis Integration With Self-Compassion

The process of self-compassion, long a feature of mystical and meditative traditions, has only recently become a focus of psychotherapeutic models, including ACT. Like mindfulness before it, self-compassion was seen as too spiritual a concept and was only grudgingly admitted to the pantheon of mental health treatments early in the twenty-first century, largely thanks to the writings of Kristin Neff (2003). Although self-compassion is not explicitly conceptualized as a therapeutic technique in her work, its clinical applications soon became obvious as research studies began to show a strong positive relationship between self-compassion and mental well-being. Trauma-exposed individuals with more self-compassion have been shown to function better in everyday life and to be less likely to attempt suicide or to develop PTSD. Similar findings have been obtained for people who experience other kinds of stress and challenge (summarized in Neff et al. 2020). The work of Paul Gilbert led to a therapeutic model called "compassion-focused therapy" (e.g., Gilbert 2014). These developments have produced an explosion of interest in the role of self-compassion as a clinical intervention with all kinds of mental health problems.

According to Neff (2003), self-compassion is about how we *relate* to the pain, just like mindfulness and acceptance. She describes three primary dimensions of self-compassion:

- Mindfulness vs. overidentification
- Self-kindness vs. self-criticism
- Common humanity vs. isolation

It's difficult to gently hold an experience in kindness while completely identifying with the experience. Thus, self-compassion involves establishing a viewpoint from which to witness the pain we are experiencing. Neff's first dimension of self-compassion is thus about mindfulness and not distinctively about self-compassion. To this calm welcoming and witnessing of experiences as they are, the second quality of self-compassion adds a caring, soothing, comforting aspect. We wrap the pain with warmth and affection. Self-compassion is not about changing negative feelings and stressful bodily states into positive and comfortable ones; it is about tenderly caring for these difficult experiences—and for ourselves while we undergo them—with kindness and love. Self-compassion means being kind to ourselves at the exact moments when we may be most likely to be harsh and self-critical. The pain of failure, loss, and fear is less a burden than our tendency to add insult to injury through an inner discourse of self-judgment that tells us we are flawed and broken and deserve to suffer. Self-compassion is beneficial in direct response to somatic stress and emotional pain, but its application to a criticized self is key to crisis integration. To treat ourselves with kindness, softness, and affection is such an important step in preventing a crisis from spiraling deeper. Finally, Neff's third dimension—common humanity—helps us recognize that we are not alone in having flaws, that our flaws join us to humanity rather than separate us. In mindfully witnessing and bringing care to experiences, we access the wider perspective that pain is part of the human experience. In moving from understanding suffering as personal ("my despair") to recognizing its ubiquity among humankind (and indeed all living beings), we can be liberated from the illusion of separation.

To embrace and care for a criticized self requires a certain amount of meta-awareness and defusion from the self-as-content, and the reverse is also true. Self-compassion itself *facilitates* movement from solidly identifying with the pain of self-rejection to knowing it from a meta-aware perspective. Although the pain is still pain, the practice of self-compassion deepens the quality of acceptance, which facilitates a self-compassionate response, and so on. Because there is no once-and-for-all escape from self-criticism, and from identification with and avoidance of experience, into self-compassion, mindfulness, and acceptance, it doesn't matter much where we begin. It is an endless process.

Marina: Clinical Dialogue on Self-Compassion

For Marina, the turnaround began when she explored ways of being mindful of her self-rejecting thoughts—for example, by waving hello to them. Marina's access to this meta-aware perspective became helpful when she was introduced to a self-compassion exercise in her next session to support her crisis integration.

Psychiatrist: How has it been going? I mean, the noticing what's going on inside?

Marina: I'm doing my best. Sometimes I can wave to the thoughts and, like, "be with" my shame, which does feel good. There's sometimes even a sigh or a deep out-breath. I like the kind of easing I get from that.

Psychiatrist: Well done for taking this on!

Marina: But it's like a drop in the ocean. Most of the time I'm still in hell.

Psychiatrist: Tell me more about life in hell.

Marina: There's nothing new really. Early mornings are worst. I think of my HIV diagnosis, and straight away I feel desperate. Then I can't get out of the idea that I'm appalling, from top to bottom.... How anyone would ever want to…

Psychiatrist: Yes?

Marina: …want to be with me? (*Starts crying.*) I just feel so shitty inside.

Psychiatrist: So on top of dealing with a very difficult situation, you're also at the receiving end of some extremely nasty judgments about yourself—like that of being appalling. (*pause*) I'm glad you have brought this up. It's something we can work with today. I have an exercise I like to use to help people explore their most difficult-to-stomach self-criticism. Are you willing to give it a try?

Marina: Okay.

Psychiatrist: Great. We'll need three chairs. You'll get to sit in all of them eventually. (*Arranges three chairs as shown in Figure 6–1.*) Let's start with this one. (*Points to a chair.*) We could call it the "self-hating chair" or the "self-critical chair." What do you think?

Marina: I don't know. "Self-critical" is maybe best.

Psychiatrist: Then we have this one over here. (*Points to the next chair.*) Here you sit when you're listening to what the one sitting in the self-critical chair is saying. Shall we call it the "hurting" or the "aching chair"?

Marina: "Hurting."

Psychiatrist: Good, the "hurting chair." We'll bring in the third chair in a little while. Okay?

Marina: Okay.

Psychiatrist: Now I'd like you to sit in the self-critical chair and say some of the harsh things you've been telling yourself for some time.

Marina: (*Moves to the self-critical chair.*) How am I supposed to do this?

Psychiatrist: Just look at the hurting chair (*Points to the hurting chair.*) and imagine that you're sitting there on the receiving end of what you're saying. Then say, "You're appalling," or whatever it is you've been telling yourself.

Marina: You're appalling. You're just appalling.

Psychiatrist: Anything else? Whatever comes.

Marina: You're sullied, appalling. Nobody will ever want to be with you. Why should they? You're a wretched, infectious, contagious loser…

Psychiatrist: Well done. Now it's time to come and sit over here in the hurting chair and let yourself receive that message. (*Marina looks at the psychiatrist as if in disbelief but moves to the hurting chair.*)

Psychiatrist: How does your hurting self feel to have heard those words?

Marina: (*Looks down.*) It just hurts so badly. I don't know what to do. What can I say?

Psychiatrist: You could say just that this hurts. Would that do enough?

Marina: (*softly*) Yes, it hurts…very much.

Self-compassionate
chair

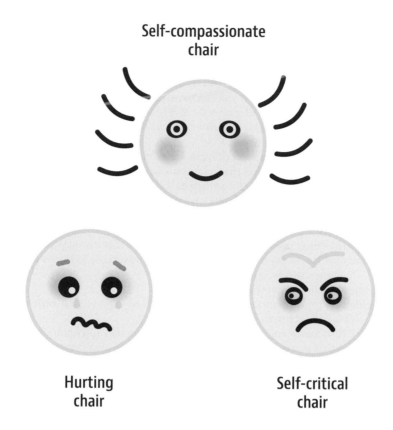

Hurting
chair

Self-critical
chair

Figure 6–1.   Chair exercise to promote self-compassion.

Psychiatrist: You'd have to be a stone for those words not to hurt.

Marina: I feel so ashamed.

Psychiatrist: I know. And shame is a really difficult emotion to be with. (*pause*) Now it's time for the third chair. We'll call it the "wise and kind chair." When you sit here, you can tap into a wise and kind part of you that's been there since the moment you were born. This part of you has been with you through thick and thin. It's eternal. It sees everything you've been through with a special clarity and is full of love for you. Would you sit here for a moment? (*Marina moves over to the wise and kind chair.*) Now I'd like to hear what you feel from the perspective of this wise and loving part of you when it looks at your hurting self.

Marina: My loving part, huh?

Psychiatrist: Yes, deepen your breath a little and see if you can connect to this loving and wise being and what she wants you to know.

Marina: (*sigh*) I feel for her.

Psychiatrist: Wonderful. Say it to the hurting chair.

Marina: Okay. (*Turns to the chair.*) I feel for you. I just want to hold you. You just need to be held.

Psychiatrist: Beautiful. Anything else she would like to say?

Marina: You hurt so much from hearing those things. There's been too much of that! I want you to feel safe and know that I'm here for you.

Psychiatrist: Wonderful. Now you can move over here again (*Points to the hurting chair.*) and tell your wise and kind self how it feels to hear those well wishes. (*Marina sits in the hurting chair and is silent a while, with her eyes closed.*)

Marina: It feels good, like something in me is relaxing.

Psychiatrist: Let yourself feel that relaxation. Scan your body to see where it's happening. Savor it for as long as you want. (*pause*) Is there anything you'd like to ask of your wise and kind self?

Marina: I want to be at peace, to get some rest, and to feel safe. Would you help me?

Psychiatrist: Move over to the wise and kind chair and see what your wise advisor has to say in response. (*Marina moves to the wise and kind chair, then suddenly looks up in surprise.*)

Marina: You know what she says?

Psychiatrist: No, I'm curious! Say what she has to say—to your hurting self—and I'll listen.

Marina: (*in a tender voice, tears rolling down her cheeks*) You know, I'm so glad that you're finally listening. I've been here all along, wanting only the best for you. I care for you deeply. (*The psychiatrist waits in silence a moment so Marina can integrate what has just shown up.*)

Psychiatrist: That's beautiful, Marina. (*smile*) Could you stay where you are for a bit? I'd like you to turn your attention to the self-critical chair. From the perspective of this wise old being, what are we to make of the self-critical part?

Marina: What do you mean, "to make of it"?

Psychiatrist: What would you imagine this self-critical part might be trying to accomplish?

Marina: That's a difficult one. Maybe it wants to help somehow?

Psychiatrist: That's an interesting idea. How about asking it?

Marina: (*addressing the self-critical chair*) Are you actually trying to be helpful by saying those things?

Psychiatrist: Move to the self-critical chair and feel your way into this part of you, to see if that's so.

Marina: (*in the self-critical chair*) I know what I say sounds mean, but I don't know what else to do. I *am* actually trying to help. I only want to protect you from more hurt. I want you to stay away from people who can hurt you.

Psychiatrist: So, this critical part is actually trying to protect you—in a backhanded kind of way. It gets you to feel so much shame that you won't risk entering the world again. (*pauses*) Marina, will you move to the hurting chair to see how it feels to be there now that you've heard from both the wise and kind and the self-critical parts of yourself.

> Marina: (*in the hurting chair*) I still feel a lot of pain, mostly sadness I think, but I feel calmer inside, more restful—and safer, more protected, than before.
> Psychiatrist: That's lovely. It sounds like connecting with that wise and kind self inside of you could be something to carry on exploring.
> Marina: I didn't know I had that in me. Yes, I will go looking for her again.

Not only had Marina felt alone in relating to her external world; she had felt desperately lonely and scared inside as a result of overidentifying with her critical self-story. In this session, she was invited to move from such identification with her harsh self-judgments (self-as-content) by taking a self-compassionate perspective (self-as-context). What also became apparent was that the "critical self" was not an internal enemy to be fought, avoided, or extinguished. It had the good intention of providing protection and was itself therefore worthy of compassion.

Through adopting a self-compassionate perspective, Marina was able to provide herself with the safety and caring she desperately yearned for. This perspective has the potential to abate the impetus toward experiential avoidance, allowing her instead to accept her inner life as well as to learn what is essential for her. Marina is by no means done with her self-critical story. It will reappear, and she will again experience loneliness, fear, and shame—and seek to avoid these feelings. But she will have firsthand knowledge that there is another road she can travel in such moments—one of choosing whether to identify with the self-critical story. The very capacity to choose will radically diminish the power of her deprecatory self-story to control her actions in the real world. What she needs to do now is to practice making this move in her everyday life. Self-compassion is something we can cultivate over time if we don't have as much access to it as we would like (Ferrari et al. 2019). The question remains: where does this competence for a caring attitude to self—as well as for others—come from?

Phylogeny and Ontogeny of Compassion

Phylogeny, the evolutionary history of a species, is informative about both the blessings and serious built-in problems of the brain. It should be kept in mind that hunting and gathering have taken up the vast majority of human history, and evolution has thus promoted competencies furthering survival in contexts quite different from those of modern times. *Ontogeny* is the development and learning within one's own lifetime, which either inhibits or facilitates those latent competencies.

Because evolution is driven by the selective replication of genes, it may at first glance be surprising that compassion should build on mental capacities that have emerged from the struggles of survival and reproduction. We have an inherited capacity for anger, fear, and behavioral avoidance that helps us manage threats to our survival—just as we have innate approach responses experienced as craving both social and material resources. If we are unaware of these latent tendencies, they can easily inhibit compassion and lead us to manage threat and reward through "hold and control" behavior in hierarchical and competitive social systems (Gilbert 2021). People then acquire a competitive mentality that reads social information in terms of power dynamics. When you are in a superior position of power, you can be exploitative and direct criticism toward others; when you are in an inferior position, criticism is turned inward. However, it is not the self-criticism itself that is the most detrimental, but the fear of exclusion and isolation (Gilbert 2019), as in Marina's acute fear resulting from the social stigma of her condition and her own perception of herself as "appalling."

Politics favoring competitive social conditions increase disparities, promote beliefs that success in life all comes down to individual striving, and boosts the fear of failing. Even successful people have a great fear of losing out (Jetten et al. 2021). Cohorts of young people in industrial countries over the past 30 years have evinced an increasing perfectionism in the form of excessively high personal standards of performance and overly critical self-evaluation (Curran and Hill 2019).

The good news is that people also have an inherited caregiving capacity that facilitates compassion, a "share and care" mentality, and egalitarian social systems (Gilbert 2021). In small hunter-gatherer communities, humans were palpably dependent on one another to survive. This interdependence promoted competencies in social interaction. Caring and sympathetic behavior was conducive to reciprocal support, cooperation, conflict reduction, and the flourishing of the group and hence of the individuals within the group. But those inherited capacities need somehow to be *facilitated*. At the present point in history, perspective-taking, care, and compassion are qualities we urgently need to awaken and cultivate on a global scale for the sake of our shared planet and the survival of our own and other species. As the Dalai Lama says, "Love and compassion are necessities, not luxuries. Without them humanity cannot survive."

There are three directions in which compassion can flow. We can receive compassion *from others*, we can experience *self-compassion*, and we can direct compassion *toward others*, including all kinds of living things (Figure 6–2) (Gilbert et al. 2011; Neff 2003).

Compassion for others involves attention to their distress and needs and a motivation to respond to these needs, whether through protection,

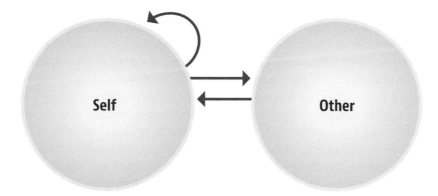

Figure 6–2.   The three flows of compassion.

nurturance, soothing, or any other expression of care (Gilbert 2014). Compassion requires collateral psychological capacities such as empathetic understanding and meta-awareness—plus motivation to care for another. Although empathy is a prerequisite for compassion, it is not the *same* as compassion. Empathy is an innate perspective-taking capacity to understand others' feelings and needs. The brain mediates an empathetic response through creating an emotional experience similar to what the other is experiencing (Klimecki et al. 2014). A canny brain-imaging study has demonstrated that when a subject believes a loved one has received a painful stimulus (an electric shock), the neural network that processes negative affect in that subject shows activity similar to that of the subject who actually receives the painful stimulus (Singer et al. 2004).

    Another aspect of compassion as an evolution-driven capacity is in how a caregiving attitude is conducive to successful childrearing. Parents provide protection, support, guidance, and encouragement, which adds up to a secure base for the child to explore and play. If the parents are also able to soothe emotions and bodily states relating to threat and desire, the child will experience a safe haven in which to rest and find comfort (Gilbert 2020). In consequence, children develop a warm attitude toward themselves and come to see other people as competent and caring. This kind of start in life facilitates self-compassion, self-reassurance, and trust in the unfolding of events, all of which are needed to face life's challenges. Although Marina had exercised self-condemnation for many years in relation to her unfortunate situation, the psychiatrist was able to elicit self-compassion from her fairly easily because Marina was able to draw on the experiences from her upbringing in which her single mother had treated her in a caring, nurturing way.

In the unfortunate case of a child who was raised by uncaring parents or who experienced abuse or neglect, their threat avoidance system may easily be activated later in life. Moreover, an impulse of craving may readily be triggered, reflecting an underlying deficit of safety, satisfaction, and sense of connection. People with this background—and the prior learning it entails—may not only have a hard time using others as a secure base and safe haven when in crisis but also not see the point of self-compassion or receiving compassion from others, because they lack this frame of reference. In responding to hardship, they tend to be harshly self-critical and to believe that they will always be alone without love, that they are unworthy of love, and that it is their own fault when they are maltreated. Encounters with compassion may even activate acute fear (Gilbert et al. 2011). Targeting this *fear of compassion* with acceptance and mindfulness will prove to be significant for crisis integration.

Crisis Integration With Acceptance of "Fear of Compassion"

Fear of compassion is implicated in PTSD, anxiety, and self-harm and is perhaps most extensively associated with depression (summarized by Gilbert et al. 2014; Merritt and Purdon 2020). Lucía, whom we met in Chapter 5, experienced all of these conditions. For patients with a background like hers, the suggestion of practicing self-compassion may elicit responses of suspicion, hostility, aloofness, and withdrawal. Such responses can be confusing to a psychiatrist, but there is a logic behind them. When childhood experiences of formative relationships have been characterized by the violation of physical and psychological boundaries, the same sense of danger can be activated in response to any reference to interpersonal closeness (Gilbert et al. 2011). To put this in terms of predictive coding, current relationships requiring some level of empathetic and compassionate interchange can evoke predictions of deceit, criticism, and abuse based on prior models of close interpersonal relations.

Such patients often regard the practice of self-compassion as silly, offensive, and, for them, unimaginable. Beneath the surface level of such thoughts and evaluations, self-compassion paradoxically evokes physical sensations of intense somatic agitation; emotions of fear, anger, grief, emptiness, and shame; and a profound sense of being undeserving and unlovable. Although the usual assumption is that self-compassion promotes warmth and caring within, it can also pull patients into quite the opposite kind of experiences. This is not an aberration limited to a small subset of patients but is, in fact, a very common response. One process goal of the practice of self-compassion is to shine the light of awareness on everything that can function as a barrier to being self-compassionate.

Should Lucía decide to take on this practice, she would benefit from gaining a greater ability to tolerate distress (see Chapter 5). Mindfulness of body and acceptance provide the interoceptive exposure needed to gain new learning about affiliative emotions of care and kindness. Acceptance of "fear of compassion" is no different than acceptance of "fear of anxiety."

Self-compassion may sound airy-fairy, but there is clear evidence that it functions as a powerful mechanism of emotional regulation. Higher levels of self-compassion correlate inversely with depression, anxiety, and PTSD symptom severity (Dahm et al. 2015; Forkus et al. 2020; Hiraoka et al. 2015; MacBeth and Gumley 2012; Neff et al. 2007). Thus, the acquisition of self-compassion skills could be expected to give Lucía significant clinical benefits.

Lucía: Clinical Dialogue on Acceptance of Fear of Self-Compassion

Lucía had been practicing mindfulness of body for some weeks in the group setting as well as at home. She had gained some proficiency in returning to her "islands of safety"—for example, her feet—when she was close to feeling overwhelmed, and she had improved her distress tolerance. However, she struggled when some phrases of self-compassion were used in a mindful breathing exercise. Lucía spoke up after the exercise to say she found the exercise to be "silly," "bullshit," and "a big waste of time" and then walked out of the group room. During the following nights, she had a hard time getting to sleep, her suicidal thoughts became more frequent and invasive, and, fearing that she might act out her suicidal impulses, Lucía went to the emergency room and asked for admission to the psychiatric unit so she would be unable to hurt herself. She was admitted to inpatient care, where the ACT group leader visited her the next day.

Psychiatrist: Hi Lucía. I'm glad to see you again, but of course I'm sure this is not what you wanted to see happen. Anyway, I'm glad you're here.

Lucía: (*Sits with arms crossed, looking down.*) Hi.

Psychiatrist: How have you been doing since Monday's ACT meeting?

Lucía: I wouldn't be here if things were going well. That's obvious, isn't it?

Psychiatrist: Yes, you're right. That's obvious. Would you tell me a little bit more about what's been going on for you? The last thing I heard you say was that you weren't getting much from the self-kindness exercise.

Lucía: Not exactly that. I said it was bullshit.

Psychiatrist: Yes, that was it. So, tell me, how did you end up here?

Lucía: I hardly ever go to the ER, but this time I just couldn't cope. I felt so angry after I attended that meeting. I felt—I don't know—more awful inside than I've felt for a long time.

Psychiatrist: It's good, then, that you came here.

Lucía: In the ACT group, I like doing the foot thing and the mindful breathing, or whatever you call it. But I don't buy this thing about being nice to yourself.

Psychiatrist: So you like mindfulness, but you didn't like the part about being kind to yourself that we did on Monday. Do you have any sense of what it is that you find "bullshit" about it?

Lucía: It was phony. Superficial. Fabricated. Like putting a fairy-tale sticking plaster on everything. That is exactly what I don't want to do, and I'm not going to.

Psychiatrist: (*pause*) I'm going to tell you a secret: I had the exact same reaction you did when I first heard about this self-kindness, or what we call "self-compassion." It just didn't make sense to me.

Lucía: Yeah? And now what? Now you've seen the light and become the guru of kindness?

Psychiatrist: (*Smiles a little.*) I sure hope not. Do you think, Lucía, that you're angry with me for talking about self-kindness, or are you angry about the *idea* of self-kindness?

Lucía: Both, I guess. (*sigh*) Well, I think I'm mostly angry about the idea.

Psychiatrist: Would it be okay for us to be for a while with your being angry about the idea of being kind to yourself? To see whether this anger has something to tell us?

Lucía: (*another sigh*) Okay.

Psychiatrist: Great, Lucía. I know this is hard, and I'm glad you're willing to try it. So, will you see now if you can make room for the anger, to welcome it, say hello to it? Can you do that?

Lucía: (*Gazes at her lap.*) Yeah, but—I don't know—it's not so much like I'm angry, I'm not sure I even *deserve* kindness. Like I told my husband: he can tell me I'm a beautiful person on the inside as much as he wants, but that doesn't mean I'm going to believe it, because I don't.

Psychiatrist: So something really powerful is showing up when it comes to being kind to yourself. Maybe anger. Maybe feeling like you don't deserve love.

Lucía: I don't know *what* is going on.

Psychiatrist: That's okay. Just stay with whatever's going on. Let it be as it is. And take a breath, or two. Maybe you could ask whatever is there if it needs anything from you—or us.

Lucía: I don't know. Maybe it wants me to take it slow.... I'm just so scared.

With the support of the psychiatrist, Lucía manages to stay present to her inner response to the idea of self-kindness long enough to investigate it. It's not strange that Lucía doesn't have many words for what is going on inside her, after having ignored the complexity of this for so long. When she begins to relate to her experience with just a tiny bit of curiosity, it reveals something of what else is going on besides anger: a sense of being undeserving of love; and there is also fear.

Psychiatrist: You can tell the fear that we'll be sure to take this nice and slow. If we start moving too fast, it can tell us again. Okay?

Lucía: I don't want to be this scared! I don't like it!

Psychiatrist: Fear is tough to stand next to. Let's see if we can give you a bit more of an anchor here. Without pushing away being afraid, move your attention around for a little while. See if you can tune into sounds you can hear in the room right now. See if you can slow down and listen to whatever shows up.

Lucía: (*Takes a breath.*) I can hear the fan, I suppose.

Psychiatrist: Good.

Lucía: Some traffic outside.

Psychiatrist: Yes?

Lucía: The clock ticking.

Psychiatrist: Good. And now, just take a peek at being afraid. How is it doing?

Lucía: Better. I just don't know why I'd be so scared.

Psychiatrist: My guess is that the anger and fear you felt in response to the self-compassion exercise have served you very well in the past. They tell you that something dangerous is about to happen. They sound the alarm, so to speak. Does this seem likely to you?

Lucía: (*quietly*) Uh-huh. "Alarm" is about right.

Psychiatrist: To be kind to yourself and to let someone else treat you kindly, you have to lower your guard a little bit. To judge by what you've told me about your family when you were growing up, letting your guard down could be dangerous. Instead of them being kind to you, and caring for you, and making you feel safe, the opposite happened. People you trusted were mean to you. They hit you. They neglected you. They criticized you and made you feel unloved. A kid in that kind of situation is going to learn to keep their guard up, to mistrust others, to try to avoid getting hurt.

Lucía: I couldn't even let myself fall asleep sometimes. I…
(*silence*)

Psychiatrist: Yes, it's hard to sleep in that kind of world.

Lucía: If the TV was on, I knew we were safe, sort of, but when the silence came, at night, it was dangerous. I'd barricade myself and my siblings in our room. Even so, Dad could come in drunk, right into our room, and start roaring around and getting violent.

Psychiatrist: So, instead of having a sober dad who would tuck you in and wish you goodnight, like fathers are supposed to do, you had to keep your guard up and not let yourself fall asleep, so that you could protect your brother and sisters?

Lucía: I had to protect them.

Psychiatrist: You had to protect yourself, and your brother and sisters as well, and you learned how to keep your guard up.

I'd guess that being mad and being afraid served you well in doing that.

Lucía: I guess I've been angry and afraid a long time.

Psychiatrist: And the anger and fear have helped you get through a lot of challenging moments. So we don't want to get rid of them; we want to respect them and listen to what they have to say. They may be signaling to you that trust and safety are things you deeply care about.

Lucía: (*Looks confused.*) Well, yes, I suppose they helped me get through tough times. But I still don't like them.

Psychiatrist: I don't like being angry or afraid either. But they are basic human feelings, and we all have them. The trick is to not let them bully you around so that you can't live the life you want to live. I imagine that you want to be close to your husband, but at the same time it's difficult for you to trust his kind words, to let his kindness touch you. Sometimes, when anger and fear show up in response to his caring for you, you may even push him away, and then anger and fear will fall away—until the next time someone tries to be kind to you.

Lucía: That sounds like the story of my life, right there.

Psychiatrist: The fear and anger are designed to protect you from getting hurt, betrayed, or let down. The flip side of them, the reason you need to protect yourself at all, is, I gather, that you care about safety and trust and, maybe, kindness. You want to be safe. You want to be close. You want to trust others. You want to be cared for. You want to receive kindness. How does that sound to you?

Lucía: That is a weird idea. Me, truly caring about being close to someone, or caring about kindness?

Psychiatrist: Try to feel your way into it; is there a place in your heart where you yearn to belong?

Lucía: I guess so, but the fear is so powerful. At the ACT group on Monday, I started shaking inside. I felt the anger well up in me, like I was going to explode. Then I had to say something, like I did, and leave. I didn't know what else to do.

Psychiatrist: And actually, that's okay too. When the feelings get intense, you can tell whoever you're with, "I need some time out." There is one other thing you could try, though, if you'd like to try something different. At the very moment when strong feelings well up inside, you could attend to the sensations in your feet—your "islands of safety"—as we've practiced. That might help you regain some of the sense of balance you need in order to be able to stay and to tolerate the inner turmoil instead of running away. It might give you the time to think about what you really care about—or maybe even to receive some kindness. Maybe that which you care about will be what guides your next actions, not the anger and fear.

Lucía: That sounds nice—in theory. I just hope I can do it.

Psychiatrist: Look at it this way. It's like having a balance scale with two bowls. In one bowl you have the response of running away or pushing away closeness, and in the other bowl you have the different response of staying and letting some kindness touch you. Each time you let somebody be kind to you—and you make room for the fear, the anger, the thought that you don't deserve kindness, or the shaky feeling inside—then you put one more feather in the bowl of experiencing some kindness. If you keep adding these feathers, one little situation at a time, the scale will eventually tip so that you can practice self-compassion more easily. Think of practicing self-compassion the way you would cultivate any other skill. It's all about practice. Are you with me?

Lucía: I think so. I guess I'm gonna need a lot of feathers. I mean, I feel like I have so much baggage to let go of.

Psychiatrist: I like that phrase, "letting go." (*long pause*) Would you have the energy to explore a little what letting go might mean, before we round up?

Lucía: Sure.

Psychiatrist: Thank you. (*Hands Lucía a pen.*) Okay, I want you to grip this pen really tight. I don't want it to slip out of your hand, or even move, while you're gripping it. Can you do that? Hold it really tight, with your hand turned upward.

Lucía: Okay, got it.

Psychiatrist: Continue to hold it tight…and keep holding it…

Lucía: Okay.

Psychiatrist: Now, without moving your arm or anything, relax your fingers completely and let the pen just rest in the palm of your hand.

Lucía: Okay. (*She opens her hand, and the pen lies still in her palm.*)

Psychiatrist: Now, what happened to your relationship with the pen when you let it go?

Lucía: What d'you mean? First I had the pen in a tight grip, and now the pen is sort of resting here in my hand.

Psychiatrist: So, now that you've let go of gripping it, you're not holding the pen tight anymore. You've relaxed your grip. But the pen didn't disappear. You can see it. You can hold it. You know exactly where it is, right? You can even put it down on the table if you want to.

Lucía: Yeah.

Psychiatrist: Letting go means you release your grip on emotions like anger or fear, or on feeling shaky inside like you're going to explode, or even on thoughts like "This is crap" or "This is dangerous because I can't trust anyone" or "I don't deserve to be treated kindly." Like the pen, they're still around. They're not going anywhere. You don't have to change them or get rid of them. You can be aware of them. You can hold them gently. And in doing this, you can even offer them a little kindness. The neat thing about letting go is that, although a decision is required to do it, it requires no effort at all. Clinging to something, on the other hand, requires a lot of effort. Simply relaxing your fingers and opening your hand is the opposite of effort.

Lucía: This is all kind of new for me. To be honest, I feel a bit disoriented. But it sounds like it's worth a try. I guess I feel more willing now to talk about self-kindness.

Psychiatrist: To treat yourself with kindness and acceptance—particularly in moments that become painful, scary, and difficult—that's what we're talking about.

In this interaction, the psychiatrist shows Lucía how acceptance and self-compassion work together. Whereas Lucía's previous model of close interpersonal relating has been characterized by danger and fear, mindfulness of body and acceptance of the fear provide the interoceptive exposure needed to gain new learning with respect to affiliative emotions.

The same theory about the benefit of distress tolerance described in Chapter 5 is thus relevant to approaching the fear of compassion. Although Lucía had previously enlarged her capacity for distress tolerance, this dialogue reveals her need for more practical guidance on how to expose herself to her full-blown fear of compassion. She is given yet another soupçon of what it could mean to allow the fear just to be (acceptance)—instead of gripping it tight, struggling with it, or reacting to it. The more that Lucía learns to accept the fear of compassion that arises from her prior learning, the more she will be able to open up to receive life-sustaining care and compassion in the present moment. Having had little experience of receiving kindness and respect during her upbringing, she has to begin by learning how self-compassion feels—the warmth, the soothing, the well-wishing—when directed toward herself. She will need to have patience, because this kind of learning is very gradual (Singer and Engert 2019). A good place for her to start could be outside the realm of people—for example, by feeling the warmth of sunrays through the whole of her being, noticing the soft evening breeze caressing her cheeks, or noticing the floor bearing her weight while she is lying down. Anything that can awaken a sense of being held, embraced, warmed, and even nurtured. At times when it proves too difficult to include herself in caring, Lucía can focus on cherishing well wishes toward a pet or anything else that it is relatively easy for her to care for. Even a stone will do. With time, the well-wishing and kindness of this practice will spill over to encompass herself and the other people in her life.

Acceptance of Avoidance

As Lucía's process illustrates, practicing self-compassion sometimes includes accepting the fear of compassion, as well as accepting any avoidance strategies relating to the fear of compassion. Likewise, acceptance of emotional pain also includes acceptance of experiential avoidance. ACT grew out of behavioral psychology that originally centered on exposure to fear. ACT has therefore emphasized acceptance—a willingness to open up to experiencing emotional pain. However, whereas early behaviorist exposure swung a sledgehammer at strategies to avoid fear, ACT brings acceptance and kindness to the experiential avoidance itself. This may seem a bit counterintuitive. Let's explain how it works.

In order to accept unconditionally, it helps to know and see clearly what you are accepting. The more open you are to what is going on inside you, the wider your acceptance can go. When you are inclined to brace against and move away from emotional pain, this too is mindfully witnessed and accepted. Paying close attention, without creating any friction with experience, rejecting nothing, saying yes to everything—even to the avoidance strategies—becomes what we call *radical acceptance*. In radical acceptance, you do not fight with or oppose yourself at any level—neither on the level of emotional pain nor on the level of avoiding such pain. As a matter of fact, it is not unusual to discover multiple layers of distress, avoidance, and self-criticism. To give a common example: you have an experience, say, of fear or restlessness, from which you distract yourself (e.g., by scrolling social media late at night). Then you add a layer of self-criticism for engaging in this distraction. This self-criticism generates another inner layer of hurt and discouragement, which you then avoid through yet more distraction—and on it goes. Although this adding of layers may seem perpetual, it is not. You can always witness with acceptance and self-compassion everything that is going on inside, and doing so will interrupt the cycle.

In a similar way, psychiatrists can help their patients adopt an accepting and compassionate attitude toward their avoidance strategies: "Of course it makes perfect sense that you'd want to avoid experiencing so much anguish." Acceptance does not mean that the psychiatrist should like, agree with, condone, or act on the patient's unviable paradigm of avoidance as a solution in crisis. But if the psychiatrist *opposes* the paradigm, they may become impatient with or even resent the patient's requests. This impatience may leak out as an attitude of "Let's get over with this validation dance as quickly as possible so we can move on to the bit where I tell you what you're doing wrong and what you should do instead."

What is profound here is that the psychiatrist has neither to act on nor get rid of their impatience; they merely have to stay mindful and accepting of it. It is the acceptance process itself that needs to be happening in the room. When psychiatrists observe and embrace any conflict and re- sistance within themselves in relation to their patients' counterproduc- tive behavior, they also support the patients' mindfulness and acceptance processes. If the psychiatrist also accepts their own inability to give the patient an instant remedy, they can similarly extend acceptance to the pa- tient's futile efforts to curtail their emotional pain. These various dynam- ics of acceptance, all interweaving with each other, thus become a very powerful clinical tool, sourced within the psychiatrist, to promote accep- tance within the patient. The patient's realizations that their experiences are being fully accepted by the psychiatrist become moments of learning what acceptance can feel like. The psychiatrist can rest assured that, when a patient's avoidance strategies are received in a spirit of acceptance that this is what is happening right now, that will not be where the story ends. Patients' learning that their experience, their experiential avoidance, and indeed themselves can all be held in acceptance and compassion sets the stage for the transformation of unviable avoidance behaviors.

Moreover, the less we struggle with any experience, or avoidance thereof, within ourselves or within others, the more we conserve valuable energy. In a time when health practitioner burnout is skyrocketing, acceptance is a key skill to build.

Acceptance, Mindfulness, Compassion, and Self-Compassion Protect Against Professional Burnout

Even before the COVID-19 pandemic, the risk of burnout was twice as high in the health care community as it was in the general U.S. working population (Shanafelt et al. 2012). The overarching problem of workload and efficiency expectations exceeding the available time and resources is an imperative organizational matter (National Academies of Sciences, Engineering, and Medicine et al. 2019). Another major contribution to burnout is the emotional exhaustion of empathizing with patients who are suffering, sometimes called "empathy fatigue" (Neff et al. 2020). If psychi- atrists instead choose to brace themselves against feeling the pain of their patients' present and past situations, they risk paying the price of becom- ing toughened and disengaged. But there is another way, and it may not come as a surprise that it involves acceptance, mindfulness, and compas- sion for others and oneself.

Acceptance and mindfulness provide an avenue by which psychiatrists can manage their personal health while engaging with the suffering of those they serve. Psychiatrists can allow themselves to fully empathize with a patient's pain and hopelessness and at the same time rest in calm meta-awareness and acceptance of the emotional distress arising inside themselves. They become less absorbed in the suffering of others, and thus less burdened by it, without closing their hearts to it. The stance of allowing the suffering to be there, as it is, without struggle or resistance, is in itself protective against fatigue.

By taking a compassionate perspective, we access the motivation to be of service. Consider one commonly overlooked aspect of compassion: the intentional development of professional skills, often taking many years of education, in order to give effective care to others. To undertake long, demanding training in a medical or other caring profession is a compassionate action in itself. At work, those of us in such professions also pay close attention to important details, and bravely make tough and quick decisions, in the service of healing and protecting those in need. When work is intense and energy is running low, we may find it difficult to access the other psychological qualities we associate with compassion—those of warm and caring concern. To try to do so feels like yet another demanding undertaking. At such times, we first need to rest. Only when restored can we aspire to embody these qualities, which not only support patients in distress but also may decrease stress responses in ourselves as caregivers (McDonald et al. 2021).

Compassion is less fatiguing than empathy for others' distress. Like mindfulness and acceptance, compassion can even be a buffer against empathy fatigue (Neff et al. 2020). Whereas mindfulness holds suffering with equanimity, compassion for others holds their distress with kindness, connectedness, and gentleness. Compassion also allows the caregiver a more positive and fulfilling experience than does mere empathy with the patient's distress. Whereas empathy activates a neural network associated with the processing of negative affect, compassionate relating activates a network associated with positive affect, social bonding, and reward (Klimecki et al. 2014).

If psychiatrists practice directing compassion toward themselves, they will be more likely to take good care of themselves *off the job*—through resting, exercising, music, and other self-nourishing activities. Also important to the health care practitioner is that self-compassion is a means to protect themselves *on the job* against the effects of stress (Neff et al. 2020). When we're in distress from not measuring up to external expectations, let alone to our own professional values when the situation is almost insurmountable, we can offer ourselves compassion. Self-compassionate professionals report less emotional and physical exhaustion, less stress and sleep disturbance, and lower levels of burnout (summarized in Neff et al. 2020). Moreover, whereas self-criticism interferes with the pursuit of goals, self-compassionate people are less afraid of failure and more likely to try again when they fail (see Kim et al. 2020; Neff et al. 2020). Self-compassion entails a kind and supportive attitude toward ourselves in times of pain, setbacks, or even failure.

All ACT Processes Are Interdependent

In sum, compassion is about kindness and soothing as well as about invigorating, courageous engagement with suffering. Although not explicitly included in Neff's definition of self-compassion, intentional action is central to Gilbert's definition of compassion as "sensitivity to suffering in self and others with a commitment to try and alleviate and prevent it" (Gilbert 2014). The "alleviation of suffering" is not to be mistaken as complicity with experiential avoidance; it refers rather to mindful and deliberately chosen action intended to change the course of development of a painful situation to the better. Compassion means the willingness to turn with kindness toward suffering in self or other, allied to the cultivation of wisdom of how best to be of service (Gilbert et al. 2019). As seen in detail in Chapter 7 ("Engagement"), the more we can orient our focus to being genuinely helpful in such a way, the more sense of purpose we will feel and the happier and healthier we shall be (see Southwick and Charney 2012).

In Chapter 4, we saw Marina mindfully recognize and verbalize her excruciating sense of loneliness, of not belonging, and her wish to be held unconditionally. With that explicit knowledge, she was motivated in her next consultation to feel fully the distress of her "hurting self" and to make the move from self-rejection to self-compassion. Although Lucía was severely depressed, she had retained a streak of curiosity and courage to explore unknown territory. In the process of expanding on her abilities to accept and mindfully tolerate distress, in this case "fear of compassion," and in connecting with her caring about emotional closeness to her family, she became willing, little by little, to learn how to receive life-enhancing kindness.

In turning toward suffering in this way, Marina and Lucía are opening up to it, accepting it, and learning new ways to care for themselves. Since there is a relationship between values and emotional discomfort, this kind of wise inward attention will help them examine their basic aspirations, needs, and values. As we see in Chapter 7, discovering some notion of the direction in which you want your life to go will expand your ability to face your pain. This back-and-forth movement is represented by the slaloming arrow between the acceptance and engagement boxes shown earlier in Figure 3–3.

It *is* without question a big task to let go of avoidance strategies in favor of acceptance, mindfulness, and self-compassion. It's not something you may feel motivated to do just because someone tells you, "It's good for you." Being clear about what is truly important to you, in a crisis or in life in general, will empower you to make room for the inner turmoil that can come with heading in a new direction. In the crisis integration model, an engagement with life on life's terms is absolutely essential.

References

Castilho P, Pinto-Gouveia J, Duarte J: Two forms of self-criticism mediate differently the shame-psychopathological symptoms link. Psychol Psychother 90(1):44–54, 2017 27249062

Curran T, Hill AP: Perfectionism is increasing over time: a meta-analysis of birth cohort differences from 1989 to 2016. Psychol Bull 145(4):410–429, 2019 29283599

Dahm KA, Meyer EC, Neff KD, et al: Mindfulness, self-compassion, posttraumatic stress disorder symptoms, and functional disability in U.S. Iraq and Afghanistan War veterans. J Trauma Stress 28:460–464, 2015

The Dalai Lama: The Middle Way: Faith Grounded in Reason. Translated by Jinpa T. Somerville, MA, Wisdom Publications, 2009

Ferrari M, Hunt C, Harrysunker A, et al: Self-compassion interventions and psychosocial outcomes: a meta-analysis of RCTs. Mindfulness 10:1455–1473, 2019

Forkus SR, Breines JG, Weiss NH: PTSD and alcohol misuse: examining the mediating role of fear of self-compassion among military veterans. Psychol Trauma 12:364–372, 2020

Gilbert P: The origins and nature of compassion focused therapy. Br J Clin Psychol 53(1):6–41, 2014 24588760

Gilbert P: Psychotherapy for the 21st century: an integrative, evolutionary, contextual, biopsychosocial approach. Psychol Psychother 92(2):164–189, 2019 30932302

Gilbert P: Compassion: from its evolution to a psychotherapy. Front Psychol 11:586161, 2020 33362650

Gilbert P: Creating a compassionate world: addressing the conflicts between sharing and caring versus controlling and holding evolved strategies. Front Psychol 11:582090, 2021 33643109

Gilbert P, McEwan K, Matos M, et al: Fears of compassion: development of three self-report measures. Psychol Psychother 84(3):239–255, 2011 22903867

Gilbert P, McEwan K, Catarino F, et al: Fears of happiness and compassion in relationship with depression, alexithymia, and attachment security in a depressed sample. Br J Clin Psychol 53(2):228–244, 2014 24283291

Gilbert P, Basran J, MacArthur M, et al: Differences in the semantics of prosocial words: an exploration of compassion and kindness. Mindfulness 10:2259–2271, 2019

Hiraoka R, Meyer EC, Kimbrel NA, et al: Self-compassion as a prospective predictor of PTSD symptom severity among trauma-exposed U.S. Iraq and Afghanistan war veterans. J Trauma Stress 28:127–133, 2015

Jetten J, Mols F, Steffens NK: Prosperous but fearful of falling: the wealth paradox, collective angst, and opposition to immigration. Pers Soc Psychol Bull 47(5):766–780, 2021 32779550

Kant I: Critique of Pure Reason (1781). Translated by Pluhar WS. Cambridge, MA, Hackett Publishing, 1996

Kim JJ, Parker SL, Doty JR, et al: Neurophysiological and behavioural markers of compassion. Sci Rep 10(1):6789, 2020 32322008

Klimecki OM, Leiberg S, Ricard M, et al: Differential pattern of functional brain plasticity after compassion and empathy training. Soc Cogn Affect Neurosci 9(6):873–879, 2014 23576808

MacBeth A, Gumley A: Exploring compassion: a meta-analysis of the association between self-compassion and psychopathology. Clin Psychol Rev 32:545–552, 2012

McDonald MA, Meckes SJ, Lancaster CL: Compassion for oneself and others protects the mental health of first responders. Mindfulness (N Y) 12(3):659–671, 2021 33204359

Merritt OA, Purdon CL: Scared of compassion: fear of compassion in anxiety, mood, and non-clinical groups. Br J Clin Psychol 59(3):354–368, 2020 32367569

National Academies of Sciences, Engineering, and Medicine; National Academy of Medicine; Committee on Systems Approaches to Improve Patient Care by Supporting Clinical Well-Being: Taking Action Against Clinician Burnout: A Systems Approach to Professional Well-Being. Washington, DC, National Academies Press, 2019

Neff K: Self-compassion: an alternative conceptualization of a healthy attitude toward oneself. Self Ident 2:85–101, 2003

Neff KD, Kirkpatrick KL, Rude SS: Self-compassion and adaptive psychological functioning. J Res Pers 41(1):139–154, 2007

Neff KD, Knox MC, Long P, et al: Caring for others without losing yourself: an adaptation of the mindful self-compassion program for healthcare communities. J Clin Psychol 76(9):1543–1562, 2020 32627192

Seth A: Being You: A New Science of Consciousness. London, Faber & Faber, 2021

Shanafelt TD, Boone S, Tan L, et al: Burnout and satisfaction with work-life balance among US physicians relative to the general US population. Arch Intern Med 172(18):1377–1385, 2012 22911330

Singer T, Engert V: It matters what you practice: differential training effects on subjective experience, behavior, brain and body in the ReSource Project. Curr Opin Psychol 28:151–158, 2019 30684917

Singer T, Seymour B, O'Doherty J, et al: Empathy for pain involves the affective but not sensory components of pain. Science 303(5661):1157–1162, 2004 14976305

Southwick SM, Charney DS: Resilience: The Science of Mastering Life's Greatest Challenges. Cambridge, UK, Cambridge University Press, 2012

Werner AM, Tibubos AN, Rohrmann S, et al: The clinical trait self-criticism and its relation to psychopathology: a systematic review—update. J Affect Disord 246:530–547, 2019 30599378

7

Engagement

Stay connected to your needs.

—Marshall Rosenberg

Three Aspects of Engagement

"We cannot solve a crisis without treating it as a crisis. And if solutions within the system are so impossible to find, then maybe we should change the system itself." This simple truth was articulated by Greta Thunberg, a young Swedish environmental activist (Rigitano 2018). Thunberg's words point in the direction of using our meta-abilities to witness our collective systems, models, and rules (see Chapters 2 and 5) and discern what works and what doesn't. If acting according to particular models will endanger many of Earth's species, including our own, then, obviously, we need to change the models.

It has been reported that as a child Thunberg became deeply troubled when she learned about the general failure to address the climate crisis (Alter et al. 2019). At age 15, she found a way to go into the world and do what was within her power to try to make the world a safe place for all living things. To act in line with her sincerely held values meant sitting outside the Swedish Parliament for 1 day a week with a sign saying, "School Strike for Climate." Thunberg's values-consistent behaviors to do something about the climate crisis grew and grew until, at age 16, she was included in *Time* magazine's list of the 100 most influential people in the world (Alter et al. 2019). The power of her message resonates with the deep anguish, anger, and despair felt by many about the world's inaction in the face of the impending climate catastrophe. Her unabashed willingness to challenge whole assemblies of world leaders serves as an example to live according to one's values rather than to please or appease anyone. In her own words, Thunberg doesn't want us to hope; she wants us to panic (Thunberg 2019), because to carry on hoping that everything will be all right can—in a crisis—be yet another way to avoid facing the difficult emotions, and hence the problem, and acting accordingly.

The climate crisis offers an excellent example of the crisis instigation model at the societal level because it hinges on large-scale avoidance and denial of what actually is going on. This allows large segments of society to disengage from any form of accountability or attempts to solve the problem (Cohen 2021; Levermann 2019). As in the ACT crisis integration model, it is only through *acceptance*—tolerating the horror and fear that climate reports ignite—and *engagement*—connecting to values of caring for and protecting all life as well as behaving accordingly—that humankind has a chance of turning this rapidly escalating process around.

It is only fitting that in the last chapter of this book we focus on the most important ACT process of all: engagement. At heart, ACT is a radical behavior therapy, and the goal of every ACT treatment session is to get the patient to try something different. Even in the midst of a crisis, this stance rings true—perhaps even more so than in other situations. In essence, when people have behaved their way into psychiatric crisis, they must behave their way out of crisis. Doing the same unworkable things over and over again is not the way to alleviate a complex life challenge. Only when people vary their behavior can they have a chance of discovering better ways to cope with or solve problems.

One inflection point is the articulation of values and needs, which, as a rule, will require some gentle, compassionate probing by the psychiatrist. It is often unclear what could bring zest into one's life again—when, for example, trauma is part of their history. Trauma is very frequent; the global prevalence of childhood sexual abuse alone is 12% (Hailes et al. 2019). If inner pain, turmoil, and confusion have often threatened to overwhelm you, your choices and behavior may for years on end have been motivated by experiential avoidance to the degree that you haven't the slightest idea what would give your life a sense of importance. Likewise, if what or whom you love has passed away, it may seem as though nothing will ever again give you enough of a motive to engage with life. Many of us, furthermore, have been told to act according to social conventions and rules of "the only way," "should," and "have to"—at the cost of shutting down our curiosity about what truly matters to us and inspires us. The question becomes: How would you even begin to figure out what you actually want in life, should your choices one day cease to be primarily guided by avoidance, attachments, and rules?

The next tipping point involves identifying behaviors that would bring about the life qualities you desire. This requires imagination: widening your view of what is possible and expanding your behavioral repertoire and accessing and improving your existing problem-solving skills when necessary.

The third challenge is to form a committed action plan that patients will carry out after leaving the clinical consultation. Simply identifying values and values-consistent behaviors does not mean much unless you act on them in a deliberate, consistent way that creates larger and larger patterns of values-consistent action over time. In ACT, this is known as "committed action." Here, at the point of interface between the patient and their life context, there is a predicament that sheds light on the emphasis on mindful being and mindful doing. Although mood and stamina do increase when one acts according to their values, those actions commonly trigger the same emotional distress that they have been avoiding all along. However, patients will now be equipped with some powerful tools (acceptance and mindfulness) that they can bring to bear instead of simply running away from any emotional discomfort. What they discover—often with the help of the ACT psychiatrist—is that emotional pain and personal values are two sides of the same coin. If you want to act according to your values, emotional pain will be part of the deal.

This chapter explores how to navigate these three critical aspects of the engagement conversation. An important prerequisite is that the psychiatrist understand the central features of values and be completely clear about what is being sought during the clinical conversation. Along the way, we examine the science underpinning the potent impacts of values-based behavior at both the individual and societal levels. Values are closely connected to prosocial and altruistic motivations that are also influenced by culture. It is difficult, if not impossible, to understand many core values without seeing how they are embedded in the patient's cultural context.

Core Qualities of Values

Many of our values are closely linked to innate needs for food, safety, and nurturance. Connecting to and acting on them are therefore intrinsically reinforcing. With the development of language, as well as nonverbal models of the world, values have been extended into other areas of meaning and purpose. As mentioned in Chapter 6, we have *non-social* needs in the category of safety and sustenance, and we have *social* needs such as connection, belonging, giving and receiving care, understanding one another, and also authenticity and autonomy. We have needs relevant to our own *development*, such as learning, creativity, and inspiration; needs relating to *internal balance*, such as rest, leisure, and spirituality; and needs pertaining to *purpose*, meaning, and contributing to life.

In the ACT framework, a value is a deeply held aspiration for our life journey. A value functions like a compass—telling us which direction we want to go. When we act in a way that is consistent with a dearly held value, we experience an intrinsic sense of reward—an increased feeling of vitality. Thus, values are a tremendous source of motivation; we become motivated to do more of the same thing that made us feel good inside. We imagine the outcome of following that value in the future, and we like the psychological taste of it. Values turn on the brain's reward centers and wake us up in a similar way as imagining feasting on a favorite dinner dish will do. However, connecting to long-term values comes with less short-term craving than does a favorite food; it brings a more profound sense of contentment. The flip side is that when a patient is in the grip of avoidance strategies, they lose contact with dearly held and intrinsically reinforcing values. What is therefore needed is a temporal space for exploring values in which decisions are left until later.

Values are both timeless and time sensitive—timeless when there is more life ahead in which the value may be applied, and time sensitive in that being aware of and acting on a value always occurs in the here and now. A value of creativity can be what we would like for this very moment or day, but we may need something completely different tomorrow, such as extending compassion to a friend in need or upholding fairness in our working team. Values depend on outer context as well as inner motivation and stamina. That said, values can also be overarching. For some, creativity may be something around which they want to orient their entire life.

Values Are Different From Rules and Strategies

In ACT, winning, succeeding, loyalty, duty, control, conformity, being nice, and so on belong to the realm of rules and strategies, whereas in the realm of values we find, for example, self-efficacy, play, freedom, participation, integrity, inclusion, mutuality, kindness, and compassion. Take a moment to savor these words one by one and notice what shows up inside you as you do.

It is when we get stuck on the level of our rules and confuse strategies with values that we get into trouble. There is no end to the benefit we get from moving our focus from rules to values. Most importantly, values enable us to access more psychological flexibility. When you connect with a value there are innumerable ways to act accordingly, whereas when you connect with a rule there is only one.

Values Are Not Goals

Values are also different from goals. *Goals* are concrete achievements or events that can be accomplished and completed. In contrast, a valued action, or "committed action" in ACT terms, is an organized and ongoing pattern of behavior in the service of a dearly held value (e.g., self-care or learning to be kind). A committed action has an intrinsically reinforcing quality, even if no tangible outcome is at stake (e.g., speaking and acting with integrity). Although values extend into the future, they are also about the immediate present. Something that is valued is valued now. We are free to act in harmony with a value, a noble intention, without attachment to the result.

Values Change the Functions of Immediate Consequences

Another powerful clinical feature of values is that, through the power of language, they can transform negative consequences into positive ones. This is critical to the process of committed action because acting on personal values is not always a feel-good exercise. Often, we must engage with inherently painful events, situations, or interactions and must stand for something. That "something" is bigger than the pain of the moment and, in fact, can define what we believe in the months or years to come. Via language, we can relate a positive consequence (acting according to a value) to a negative consequence (emotional discomfort) in such a way that the meaning of the negative consequence is permanently altered. Yes, there will be moments of mounting anxiety or waves of mourning what is lost; this is part of the process of moving in the valued direction. Instead of being taken as a signal that you are doing something wrong, feelings of fear, pain, or sorrow can become understood as a signal that you are acting in line with your values. The conversion of short-term negative consequences into signals that a positive behavioral event has occurred dramatically increases the likelihood that the valued behavior will persist over time, despite any negative consequences that appear along the way.

Values and Reward Prediction Errors

Chapter 5 ("Mindfulness of Body and Feeling") described the prevailing predictive coding hypothesis of how the brain goes about the task of perception, particularly that of *interoception*, or the sense of what is going on inside the body. In short, perceptual model-based learning makes use of predictive coding algorithms: prediction errors (the mismatch between predictions based on prior knowledge and present events) are used to update prior perceptual information. In a similar manner, the brain employs learning through "reward prediction errors" to update predictions regarding rewards and to improve decision-making. In the real world, both supervised learning (in which correct answers are provided) and unsupervised learning (in which no feedback is available) are rare situations. Instead, animals and humans alike learn how to achieve what is valued mainly through rewards (i.e., things that contribute to our well-being) and punishments (i.e., things that give rise to a nasty experience). The motivation to act is not induced only in direct interaction with the environment, as in inflexible, model-free, stimulus-response learning. Both humans and some animals can also construct rich associative models of the world that can flexibly produce motivation in the absence of direct experience. In such adaptable, model-based learning, a behavioral choice is often made by simulating many possible consequences and selecting the response associated with the most favorable outcome. In other words, when we construct an action plan, we use mental models containing information about present contextual cues, what is valued, various possible actions, and the long-term consequences of our actions (Collins and Cockburn 2020; Nasser et al. 2017).

Recent neuroscientific evidence suggests that dopaminergic prediction error signals support not only model-free learning but also such model-based learning (Collins and Cockburn 2020; Nasser et al. 2017; Schultz 1997). We get a reward signal merely through *anticipation* of a future reward (e.g., Iigaya et al. 2020). To contact one of our values and imagine acting in line with it is rewarding in and of itself. Many ACT values-based interventions engage the patient in what amounts to a mental rehearsal of anticipated actions, often having the patient recall a time in the past when such actions actually occurred. This is thought to help prime the patient's motivation to act in line with what is being planned, thus increasing the likelihood that those actions will actually be undertaken.

That said, we all know that it takes resolve and persistence to mentally simulate and infer values and outcomes that go beyond merely responding to cues linked to immediate rewards (e.g., "I will feel better afterward if I close my eyes and rest for a while instead of becoming absorbed in social media on my phone"). The mental effort required to overcome what is habitual or imposed by present cues in the environment is a huge factor in crisis integration. Reduced values- and model-based control is considered to be a transdiagnostic feature in many forms of psychopathology (Voon et al. 2017). It is therefore helpful in clinical work to apply multiple strategies (e.g., mental rehearsal, experiential exercises, metaphorical communications, analogies) when trying to prime the motivational pump of personal values as incentives for the patient's actions.

Values Are Linked to Prosocial Behaviors

Trusting the internally reinforcing quality of people's values as guides for action builds on the assumption that most human beings want to be helpful, rather than harmful, both to themselves and to others. Although at times we make choices that serve ourselves alone, we feel an inherent resistance to having our needs met at the expense of someone else's. This resistance increases with greater ability to take another person's perspective.

Marshall Rosenberg, who developed Nonviolent Communication, took this one step further, arguing that if we pay close attention inward, as we do in mindfulness, we notice that our needs for safety and sustenance, for example, are not truly met until everyone is safe and has food on their table (Rosenberg M, International Intensive Training, Switzerland, 2001). In everyday language, "needs" usually connotes a self-focus, whereas "values" entails a bigger picture, but the two concepts are closely aligned in the exploration of engagement in ACT.

Are we willing to bear the cost of helping and giving to another, such as a stranger, without gaining any personal benefit? Experimental evidence supports the premise that such altruism can be, in and of itself, the force behind so-called prosocial behavior. Certainly, people's concern for others varies greatly, and if those who express selfish or even psychopathic traits are not reproached, they can undermine others' altruistic intentions. Nevertheless, altruism exists in the general population and extends far beyond kin-driven altruism (supporting beings with similar genes), reciprocal altruism ("I'll scratch your back if you'll scratch mine"), and reputation-based altruism (motivated by the opportunity to gain a reputation for being generous and helpful) (Fehr and Fischbacher 2003).

When one encounters another in need, it's compassion that drives the impetus to be helpful—even if it carries a cost—and that activates key regions in the brain associated with reward-processing, social attachment, and caregiving (FeldmanHall et al. 2015; Harbaugh et al. 2007; Zaki and Mitchell 2011). People with greater interoceptive sensitivity (see Chapter 5) have been shown to be more altruistic, which suggests that you really can "listen to your heart" to guide your altruistic behavior (Piech et al. 2017). It has even been shown that people who spend money to benefit others report more happiness (Aknin et al. 2020) and that one's ability to learn an association between actions and outcome is reinforced not only by a self-relevant rewarding outcome but also when an unknown person is the recipient of what is given (Cutler et al. 2021). The warm glow of giving, which even can be detected in toddlers (Aknin et al. 2012), is likely to relate to the satisfaction of core human needs of connection and the power to make a difference (Dunn et al. 2014). Crucially, in the context of crisis, ethical intentions and behaving to benefit others have consistently been linked to better physical and mental health and a greater sense of satisfaction in life (Alim et al. 2008; Cutler et al. 2021; Feder et al. 2016; Isaacs et al. 2017; Schaefer et al. 2013; Southwick and Charney 2012; Tsai et al. 2015; Wang et al. 2020).

In her *New York Times* bestselling book *Grit*, Angela Duckworth (2017, p. 143) described the pivotal assets that enable us to keep going when we face difficulties:

> Interest is one source of passion. Purpose—the intention to contribute to the well-being of others—is another. The mature passions of gritty people depend on both.... [T]he more common sequence is to start out with a relatively self-oriented interest, then learn self-disciplined practice, and, finally, integrate that work with an outer-centered purpose.

In crisis, when the basis of our life as we have known it becomes fragmented—when that which is closest to our hearts has been lost, whether gradually or suddenly—we naturally experience a sense of emptiness inside as well as confusion about what is important to us. Not only has the sense of meaning of our life—our beliefs about coherence, order, fairness, identity, and why things happen—been shattered, but the sense that our life has a purpose also is swept away (Park 2010). In a crisis consultation, what may ultimately carry the day is to help the patient reconnect with a sense of intentionality and purpose.

It is vital here to spell out the precarious situation that will arise when the imperative to help others and to behave like a saint is a rule the patient had to apply as a child in order to earn safety and love. In such cases, the patient first needs to open up inwardly to learn about their self-oriented needs, values, and interests, and the limits of their energy, before they engage with altruistic values. Important to their engagement process is both acceptance of the shame and fear that arise when they say yes to their own needs *and* remembering that it is just as purposeful, rewarding, and gracious to care for oneself as it is to care for another.

Values Are Nested in Cultural Contexts

In ACT, a value is not a socially inculcated rule or norm the patient must follow; to act according to their values—to what matters to them—is a free choice made solely by the patient. This is particularly important to consider with regard to the many societies in the world that have a strong communal aspect. In such communities, the individual's choices are always influenced by the norms of community and family regardless of educational level and social class. Responsibilities to the community take precedence over the individual's values. Thus, if we were to say "Tell me what's important to you," we would get answers about what is important to the group (see, e.g., the case of Yasmine later in this chapter). In societies in which *honor* is an extremely important norm, it will be accompanied by certain rules of behavior and often, when those rules are broken, by severe punishments to right the wrong, especially for women. If we probe for values upstream of honor, we will find ones of safety, belonging, and the like. Thus, honor-related rules may meet the needs of safety and belonging of some members of the community, but they paradoxically may endanger and exclude other individuals and their families. For our rules and actions to truly contribute to a value such as safety, we must check whether they contribute to the safety of *everyone* in the community. Even in an individualistic culture, you needn't go far before you stumble across rigid and constricting codes of conduct in congregations, companies, parties, gangs, clubs, teams, families, classes, and so on. Society requires some rules in order to function and provide safety, but we must examine whether those rules favor the whole of society over its parts, or the few over the larger group, and whether they are compassionate and wise with regard to everyone.

Identifying Values and Needs

Identifying values requires an active connection with personal values and life purposes. As easy as it sounds, learning about your values is—like the skills of mindfulness and acceptance—a lifelong treasure hunt. But how *do* you learn about what you need or value at this moment in time, and for your life? How are psychiatrists to know whether what the patient says is important to them is really so important? For a value to be a reliable source of motivation, it must be something honestly owned by the patient and not just something they are doing to comply with a norm, to please others, or to obtain approval (Barney et al. 2019). Long-practiced habits of attachment, avoidance, and rule-governed behavior can make it difficult to get to know your priorities.

Yasmine: Clinical Dialogue on Values and Needs Identification

Yasmine is a 30-year-old who, having moved to a new country, has learned a new language, found a job, and developed a long-term intimate relationship, which ended abruptly 2 years ago. Since the break-up, Yasmine has found it hard to get out and date again. She has admitted to her parents that she feels very lonely. In response, her father has repeatedly asked her to come back to her country of birth and marry a man of the family's choice. Her parents are coming to visit in 1 week, as they do every year. Accompanied by a friend, Yasmine turns up in the psychiatric emergency room because of her escalating panic, insomnia, and suicidal thoughts.

Psychiatrist: I understand from your admission note that your parents are coming to visit you, and that is putting a lot of pressure on you. Can you tell me a bit more about what them coming to visit is bringing up inside you?

Yasmine: My father just won't stop trying to persuade me to go back home with them. Every day he questions my decision to move here and mocks the life I'm living. And, you know, I do find it difficult to explain to him why I should stay. I'm very lonely; I'm single, and I don't have many friends. My father knows that I am not very enthusiastic about my job. I honestly find it quite boring. I don't know what I'm doing with my life!

Psychiatrist: And if you imagine going along with your father's suggestion of returning home, what comes up for you then?

Yasmine: I would, for sure, have company all day long. Every step I took and every choice I made would have to be adjusted to my family's expectations. I can barely breathe when I think of it…(*Looks down to her lap and speaks with a faint voice.*) At the same time, I love my parents very much. I know they want the best for me, and I do want to show them my respect and love. I just don't know who I am any longer, or what I should do, or even what I want to do.

Psychiatrist: That sounds like a very difficult situation to be in. It sounds like you're being squeezed between two very different cultures. One emphasizes the importance of family and close social ties; the other emphasizes being able to make it on your own and forming your own social networks.

Yasmine: That's exactly it!

Psychiatrist: And, right now, you're not really very happy with either of these options.

Yasmine: No, I'm not happy…. If my father knew that I'd come to see you, he would say, "I told you so." I just feel so confused.

Psychiatrist: This *is* a very difficult situation. No wonder you feel confused and are looking for a way out. Who wouldn't? So, let's see, might there be another angle we could pursue here?

Yasmine: (*Looks up.*) What would that be?

Psychiatrist: What if, just for a moment, you set aside the pull from different cultures and other people's expectations of you and just explore what is important to *you*, what *your* values are? Who or what matters to you right now in your life, and what kind of life would you like to live if you could choose?

Yasmine: I've already told you: I don't know what I want!

Psychiatrist: Well, maybe we could start by looking at what you *don't* want, and work backward toward what you *do* want. One thing I heard you say was that you find it difficult to breathe when you think about having to adjust to your family's expectations. Did I hear that correctly?

Yasmine: Yes, the way they see the role of women—and especially women as members of a family—is really hard to accept.

Psychiatrist: Would it be fair to say that you value your sense of freedom to make the choices you want to make in your life?

Yasmine: Yes, I do. Very much.

Psychiatrist: So you definitely value your autonomy, your freedom to make choices based on what you want, not what somebody else wants?

Yasmine: Yes.

Psychiatrist: I also hear that you care deeply about your parents and have a genuine wish to honor and cherish them.

Yasmine: Yes, that used to be my main guiding principle in life. It still is in some ways.

Psychiatrist: I understand. And you mentioned that you feel lonely, which I guess means that, like most of us, you care about closeness to other people? Maybe having a life partner, friends you can hang out with, that type of thing?

Yasmine: Yes, very much so.

Psychiatrist: Good. You also said you felt bored at your job. Even though you probably are glad to have the independence that the paycheck gives you, your boredom could mean that you'd like a different kind of job, one that means more to you.

Yasmine: Yes, I feel like I'm in a rut at work, even though I get paid pretty well. I'm not gaining new skills or feeling very challenged. It's an easy job, but it's very boring.

Psychiatrist: So let's go back to where we started, when I asked you who and what matters to you. We've developed a shortlist of things that matter to you. I'd like to see if you can expand on it for a few minutes. Just imagine that anything is possible and you're free to consider anything that's important to you in your life. You can use this list as an inspiration. (*Hands over the list of values.*) Read each item aloud and notice which ones touch your heart. Let these items spark your own phrases. You may feel drawn to, say, the value of "autonomy," which might spark your own phrase—say, "Yes, I want to make my own decisions." The values of "belonging and intimacy" may in your words become "Yes, I want to feel close to others" as well as "I have a profound desire to cherish and honor my parents." And the value of "contribution" may for you mean, "Yes, I want my work to make a true difference." In other words, you express your chosen values in your own words to see how well they fit you. Right now, you don't need to consider making any big decisions in life. Just look inward and see who and what matters to you right now. When you've got a sense of what values fit you, write them down here, in your own words. (*Hands Yasmine a blank piece of paper.*) While you do that, I'm going to go see another patient. I'll be back in about half an hour and we can go over this together to see what inspires you.

After the allotted half hour, the session continued.

> Psychiatrist: How did it go?
> Yasmine: (*Hands over the paper.*) My life seems not to be so empty of meaning as I thought. There are things I want that I don't have right now, like a partner and *more* friends. (*Looks up and gives her friend an appreciative little smile.*) But I haven't really been making an effort. I've just not done enough to get my social life going.
> Psychiatrist: Many of us, you know, have that experience of not really acting on what matters to us. Life just kind of numbs us out, and we stop paying attention. You are not alone.
> Yasmine: Well, I think I know now what I need to do with my parents. Every morning during their visit, I'm going to read this sheet again and remind myself of what I really care about. Maybe that will make me feel less desperate when my father puts the pressure on.
> Psychiatrist: That sounds like an excellent plan to me. Go for it! And know that you're always welcome back here if you need any more help.

Yasmine's acute suicidality lifted when she found a way to articulate her own values in this consultation. It placed her emotional discomfort in a different context, one that did not immediately require her to engage in such an extreme form of avoidance. In this interaction, the psychiatrist used a few practical strategies to help Yasmine make direct contact with her values. The first involved using the uncomfortable emotions she described as a pathway to reveal her unmet needs. For example, her sense of suffocation may be related to her need for a sense of autonomy so she can make decisions based on her own personal values and desires rather than on cultural prescriptions of how women should behave.

When patients in crisis don't know what is going on inside them—and frequently they don't—carefully worded suggestions from the psychiatrist can help them look inward in a productive, mindful way. The situation is comparable to trying to describe the taste of an exquisite cheese when you've never had much experience of expensive cheeses. If you are offered words such as "nutty," "barnyardy," or "fruity," you can check whether each word fits, or not, with what you are tasting. Similarly, a patient can take the words offered by the psychiatrist to refer to feelings, body sensations, needs, and values and test whether they fit. Whether the answer is a "yes" or a "no," the psychiatrist's suggestion nudges the patient to open up and observe their inner life. If the patient says "yes" to what is suggested even if it doesn't exactly fit what's going on for them, the psychiatrist will notice that the connection hasn't happened yet and may continue to probe by offering somatic, feeling, need, or value words in the hope of finding a better match. The patient may also let the psychiatrist know that "No, it's not like that, it's like this." Even if they speak in an irritable tone—frustrated by the psychiatrist missing the mark—the suggestions will have supported their inner exploration. When the psychiatrist makes suggestions, they should also make it clear that they are open to the patient's alternative responses and that the patient's "no" is welcome.

When investigating what the patient might be needing, it is important to probe for any inner experiences that might provide a clue. Random thoughts, memories, somatic sensations, urges to act in some way, and emotions in the moment, when all taken together, provide a rich tapestry. The clarification of needs and values not only will help the patient learn about their inner response to the crisis situation, what is important to them, and in which direction they want to head but will also provide a space of mindfulness as they stop and look inward. This creates an empathetic connection within the patient as well as between the psychiatrist and patient.

Holding inner experiences in *mindfulness* and *acceptance* allows one to know them better. Once the patient has recognized these experiences, they can move on to *engagement* and relate them to specific unmet values or needs. For Yasmine, the first step involved accepting and articulating her feelings of anxiety, panic, and loneliness. She then identified the values underpinning her emotional discomfort to be independence, autonomy, social connection, and intimacy. Emotional discomfort is a signal that some underlying value or need is deeply held and not being met. To just get rid of emotional discomfort is akin to putting duct tape over the "check engine" light in your car because the sight of the warning light upsets you. As Yasmine's case demonstrates, connecting unpleasant experiences with personal values changes the function of those unpleasant experiences from something that is harmful and needs to be avoided to something that is highly informative and clinically impactful.

If raising the question of who and what matters to a patient triggers an immediate defensive response, the psychiatrist can also interpret this as a request for help with some need the patient has. The patient who declares "I can't stand this" is looking for reassurance that it is okay to lean into emotional discomfort one bit at a time and that the psychiatrist will be there for them as the experience unfolds. Someone who says "Nobody understands what it's like to be me" may be asking for empathetic validation paired with compassion and acceptance. "I am just so scared" may express a need for some form of predictability, respect, or boundary setting. One who states "I'll never find a way out of this" or "I'll never make it on my own" is indicating a need for companionship when the going gets tough—and reassurance that they have what it takes to manage and solve problems, one at a time.

The next tool the psychiatrist made use of was the list of needs and values that he gave to Yasmine (see Table 7–1). From that list of prototypical value statements, Yasmine can personalize the values examples to formulate specific qualities she wants to prioritize in her life. In engagement-oriented consultations, such a list can facilitate the patient's own discovery of what they are missing and would like more of. It also helps distinguish between values and needs, on the one hand, and social rules and strategies and others' expectations, on the other. In sum, the list provides the patient with ideas and inspiration and clarifies what values and needs actually are, should the patient be unaccustomed to understanding motivations from this perspective.

Values identification entails learning about one's priorities and understanding that sometimes values conflict. In any given moment it may not be possible to act on the basis of two conflicting values, such as community and autonomy. The choice at one moment in time to follow one value rather than another does not necessarily invalidate the value that is not followed. It is possible to endorse many different values. However, Yasmine's situation illustrates a different type of quandary. Because choosing is integral to operationalizing values, it may be problematic to live in a community or family in which individual choice is highly constrained. If Yasmine were to choose to act on her value of belonging and honoring her parents' wishes by going back to her family and letting them choose her husband, she would be giving up the opportunity to make many other future choices based on her own intrinsic motivations. If she chooses to act on her value of autonomy, then, as time unfolds, she will likely have many other opportunities to choose to act on her value of cherishing her parents. The treasure hunt of identifying our values and determining priorities is intricate and ongoing. It is always a worthwhile pursuit, and in crisis it is imperative. As Yasmine's case demonstrates, some life crises are intensified, or even caused, by our not fully knowing our values.

Identifying and Commitment to Values-Consistent Behaviors

Merely connecting to one's values is not enough by itself to carry the day for most patients in crisis. Values can become displeasing, or even demoralizing, when we do not act on them. Patients in crisis are often not only clueless about what their most dearly held values are but also paralyzed

Table 7–1.   Examples of needs/values and valued behaviors

Needs/values	Valued behavior
Autonomy	To act according to my own authentic values and internal motivation.
Belonging	To build affinity, warmth, and ties with others.
Compassion	To listen to those who are suffering and act with kindness, concern, wisdom, and care to the best of my ability.
Connection	To find and experience reciprocal understanding based on respect and friendliness. To know others and allow myself to be known. To have my experience of events perceived, validated, and comprehended by others and to do the same for them. To help and be helped by others.
Creativity	To create and innovate using my own imagination. To make space in my life for creative activities. To participate in creative communities of people.
Consistency	To choose and act in ways consistent with my values. To create a sense of order.
Curiosity	To explore and discover with an open mind.
Gratitude	To express appreciation and joy for what is given.
Grieving	To mourn who or what is lost. To make room for mourning when values and needs are not met. To feel and accept sadness.
Integrity	To stand up for and speak what is true, honest, and useful. To have reverence for all living things, including other people and myself.
Intimacy	To open up and share with others that which matters most to me. To share physically intimate touch.
Learning and growth	To learn to let go of avoiding or clinging to experiences and instead accept and embrace them with compassion. To learn about my values. To acquire abilities that help me engage with what is important for me and others. To gain new understanding of myself, others, and the world.
Love	To offer and receive empathetic understanding, compassion, care, tenderness, kindness, and gratitude. To celebrate, mourn, and share each other's joys and sorrows. To provide and receive support for one another's needs and values.
To matter	To make a positive difference for others.
Mutuality	To build relationships in which the balance between giving and receiving feels fair and sustainable.
Patience	To wait calmly with trust in life's unfolding.

Table 7–1.   Examples of needs/values and valued behaviors *(continued)*

Needs/values	Valued behavior
Peace, rest, and ease	To let go of struggling with experience as it is and instead make peace with this moment, myself, and others. To let go of "doing and thinking" sometimes and make choices that nourish and calm the body, emotions, and mind.
Persistence	To continue resolutely despite difficulties.
Play and pleasure	To do things that bring enjoyment, fun, inspiration, and pleasure. To act, speak, and move light-heartedly and without unnecessary constraint. To appreciate humor.
Purpose	To act in service of the needs, values, and flourishing of other people, myself, and the world.
Safety and sustenance	To ensure that others and myself enjoy safety, protection, and nourishment.
Support	To receive and give instrumental help and compassionate understanding.
Touch	To receive and give touch that feels safe and nourishing.

by indecision over what to do. Let us, therefore, outline what will help guide patients in the direction of acting on their values.

Identifying Values-Consistent Behaviors

Yasmine finds herself compelled to engage with her pressing life situation. Non-action is not, for her, an option, as it is usually not during a crisis. She is at a crossroads in her life, and she must head down one road or another. She alluded to the fact that she has not done enough so far to bring into existence the social world and intimate relationship for which she longs. If she returns for a follow-up visit, the psychiatrist will help her list any actions she can think of that could possibly be in accord with her values of belonging and intimacy. During such brainstorming, patients should be encouraged to let go of all judgments about the ideas that come up (Nezu et al. 2013).

When trying to solve real-life problems, we need to facilitate the flow of ideas. Yasmine could, then, conjure up *any* ideas, however absurd they might initially seem to her, knowing that she would not be obliged to carry out any of them just because she had articulated them. Clearly, she does have the option to go back to her country of origin, but because she has shifted her primary focus from fixed strategies to values, she has access to options other than either moving back to the home country or staying and enduring her loneliness. She could consider reaching out and inviting colleagues for dinner or joining a choir or a hiking club. She could also consider opening up more to others. She could, for example, share her present predicament with people she trusts. This would likely create more intimate connections with a select few friends. At some point in this brainstorming phase, she will probably come across the idea of entering the dating scene, which for many people is not an easy experience. For Yasmine it might prove to be even more difficult because she would have to deal with the emotions that come with breaking previously learned cultural norms, in this case regarding women's conduct. She would not be alone, however, in encountering apparent barriers to putting ideas into action. All forms of engagement usually bring up emotional or sociocultural barriers as well as reactions linked to prior learning. Ironically, it is often the values-based action to which we are most resistant that proves to be the most fruitful. This is no coincidence; experiential avoidance and rule-based behavior regarding some pivotal aspect of life are often significant contributors to crisis.

Commitment to Values-Based Behaviors

Yasmine needs to commit to act on one or several choices that are consistent with her values and then to pay close attention to the results of these new behaviors, with the aim of revising her strategies in order to increase their effectiveness. Such active engagement in values-consistent behavior requires the navigation of any real or self-perceived barriers. If she makes herself available for dating, Yasmine will probably have to learn how to stay compassionately present to wave after wave of discomfort as she lets go of her prior learning and rules. What will support her, however, is the inherently rewarding experience of values-consistent behavior.

Mindful Doing—Staying Mindful During Engagement

Mindfulness and acceptance facilitate the first step of becoming more familiar with our values, but these capacities are just as relevant to the succeeding step in engagement—that of committed action. As we have seen, a commitment to engage in behavior that reflects personal values requires a willingness to accept and stay with the emotional agony or inconvenience that may ensue. This readiness builds on the rewarding quality inherent to connecting to our values and undertaking committed action. Yasmine could, for example, remind herself why she is opening up to dating, connect to her value of intimacy with someone, and sense how rewarding that would be as a counterfoil to the anxiety of making herself vulnerable to the uncertainties of forming new relationships, as well as of breaking the cultural norms of her upbringing. By staying mindfully aware of her personal values, she can more fully experience these values' appetitive quality. This will help her to sustain value-consistent behavior over time and in different situations. She can look beyond the immediate consequences of her actions, such as the emergence of difficult thoughts, feelings, and sensations, and stay true to the values she has prioritized.

Kai: Clinical Dialogue on Identifying and Committing to Values-Based Behavior

To illustrate another way to promote active engagement, we now return to the session with Kai that we introduced in Chapter 2 ("The ACT Model of Crisis Instigation"). Kai's engagement with life came to a grinding halt after he was defrauded by a business associate and lost everything he valued in his life, including his long-term girlfriend. He now experiences anxiety that rises to monumental levels when he tries to go out into the world or even when he thinks about doing so. His first priority has been to keep his emotional discomfort under control, a focus that has made him unable to pursue values-based action. This approach of "avoid at all cost" has produced the profoundly negative consequence of a whole new set of problems: Kai's sense of self-worth has cratered, and his future life now seems devoid of any potential meaning.

There are many worthwhile routes the psychiatrist might explore in this consultation. Kai could be guided to gradually accept more of his fear, anxiety, and sense of loss rather than automatically try to shut down these feelings when they show up. He could then be introduced to mindfulness training to see if his tolerance of distressing somatic sensations—such as heart palpitations—could be expanded. When Kai harshly blames himself for all of his losses, the psychiatrist might introduce self-compassion as an alternative to self-loathing. At the transition point in this session, however, the psychiatrist chooses to explore if Kai's almost complete disengagement from any meaningful pursuits in life might be turned around. The way to motivate Kai to reengage with his life will likely be to encourage him to connect with his values and undertake a series of committed actions, however small.

> Psychiatrist: May I ask you something else that might seem a little weird, given what you're going through?
> Kai: Okay.
> Psychiatrist: Besides the things we've been talking about—being cheated, losing your money and your business, losing your life partner, feel-

ing isolated from friends, having these daily battles with anxiety and reliving the past—is there someone or something that matters to you? Someone or something that you care about?

Kai: What do you mean, "that I care about"? I don't have anything now that makes life worth living.

Psychiatrist: Then how about before all this stuff happened to you? Who or what mattered to you when your life was going better?

Kai: Well, yeah, I cared about a lot of things, but all that's gone now. Girlfriend gone. Friends gone. Work gone. Everything is gone! Why do you figure I'd find anything important now?

Psychiatrist: Back then, it sounds like you cared about intimacy. You had a girlfriend who mattered a lot to you.

Kai: But she left me. Said I was a downer to be around because I couldn't get over being cheated out of everything.

Psychiatrist: Yes, I realize that must have been a huge blow for you emotionally. And you mentioned that you lost contact with your friends. Did those friendships matter to you—I mean, did it bother you when you lost contact with your friends?

Kai: Damn right it bothered me! But I did it to myself, I guess. Stopped going anywhere when my girlfriend left. I blame myself for that.

Psychiatrist: And I guess you were proud of the success of your business and the money you were able to save, that was important to you too?

Kai: It was my life's dream to have my own business. I used to love going to work. It felt like a challenge every day, but I felt good about it. Still can't get over what that son of a bitch did to me. And I chickened out when it came to doing something about it. I was just a loser in the whole deal.

Psychiatrist: So you were really invested in your work; it energized you and challenged you at the same time. As we talk about the things that mattered to you before this trouble descended into your life, what comes up inside for you?

Kai: (*Sits silent for several seconds.*) I feel uncomfortable. Where are you trying to go with this? (*Lowers voice.*) I just feel so ashamed of myself.

Psychiatrist: So, shame shows up?

Kai: Why's that a surprise? Of course I'm ashamed. All my friends now have a partner, children, a nice place to live, and a job. And here I am, barely able to get myself to an appointment with my shrink.

The conversation has become delicate. When the psychiatrist probes for values, Kai responds as if he is being judged for not living a meaningful life right now. He has a wish to engage in life in a similar way to how he did before he was defrauded, but with the passing of time his ideal life of a gratifying job, a loving relationship, and family of his own seems ever more beyond reach. His life, in his view, is nowhere near what it should be. For Kai, as for many patients dealing with great loss, the image of the ideal life he was seeking now stands in the way of doing anything at all.

Kai's somewhat idealized image of what his life should look like resembles what in ACT are known as "goals"—as distinct from his core values, which have not changed despite his multiple losses. His now seemingly unattainable life goals no longer motivate him to tolerate the anxiety entailed in moving on with his life. Moreover, besides being disheartened by all that he's lost, Kai blames himself, and this triggers his feeling of shame.

To sustain rapport with him, the psychiatrist now shifts the conversation to acceptance and mindfulness by gently prompting Kai to take an interest in his discomfort. Rather than offering words of encouragement or saying there is no reason to feel ashamed, she invokes an outlook of curiosity toward this feeling.

> Psychiatrist: Right now, is shame in the room?
> Kai: I'm not sure about right now. It was there just a bit ago. I felt ashamed when you asked me about important stuff in life.
> Psychiatrist: When you're reminded of the things that mattered to you, and when you compare your friends' lives with yours and see what they have and you don't, then, besides acutely missing those things, you also feel ashamed about not having them?
> Kai: Yes, I do.
> Psychiatrist: So, on top of dealing with the devastation of having lost everything dear to you, I gather that you also blame yourself for that. Like you've done something bad, something really dreadful, and maybe you deserve the life you're living right now?
> Kai: Something like that might be going on. I feel like this is all my fault, but I can't seem to get out of the rut I'm in.
> Psychiatrist: How about if you invite shame into the room right now so we can investigate it and get to know it a little better? Maybe see it in a different light?
> Kai: "Investigate"? What the hell does that mean? Shame is a horrible feeling. We don't want to investigate that!
> Psychiatrist: Well, the idea would actually be to spend some time with shame. To see if it has something to tell you. Can we try that together, right now?
> Kai: (*shrug*) If that's what you want. You're the boss.
> Psychiatrist: Are you truly willing to give it a try?
> Kai: Alright, okay.
> Psychiatrist: Good. Now, we know that thinking about how well your friends are doing in life is one trigger for shame to show up. Does any particular friend spring to mind?
> Kai: James—or Jim for short.
> Psychiatrist: Jim, great. Can you imagine watching a football game at his house? Would you be able to do that? You can close your eyes if that makes it easier.

Kai: I don't want to watch football at his place. He would ask me how I've been doing, and I would tell him my life sucks. Then he would tell me about his kids, his job, his wife, and all the fun they're having.

Psychiatrist: So shame is definitely in the room now, right? I can see it in your face. Your body looks tight and tense. Does this feel familiar to you?

Kai: You bet. It's with me all the time.

Psychiatrist: I know that shame is difficult to be with, so if you feel a pull to think about something else, will you just notice the pull? See if you can breathe in and out for a few seconds. I'll do it with you. See if you can focus on just being here with me. Just you, me, and the shame right now, Kai.

Kai: (*Takes a few breaths and then looks up at the psychiatrist.*)

Psychiatrist: Yes, the shame is welcome here. If you're going to get to know the shame a little better, then we need to welcome it into the house. At this point I'm curious: does the shame have anything to tell you about what to do about it?

Kai: What? (*Looks perplexed.*) Does the shame have anything to tell me about the shame?

Psychiatrist: What does the shame want you to do before it will agree to ease off on you?

Kai: If I understand your question, my shame wants me to sit down, shut up, and disappear. Then it won't torture me so much.

Psychiatrist: And you've done that very well, very courageously, for the past 7 years, wouldn't you say?

Kai: Yeah, I've pretty much stopped living.

Psychiatrist: Would you say the shame has kept up its end of the bargain? I mean, how many years do you have to spend in exile? When is the shame going to let you off the hook? Or should I say, when will you unhook yourself from shame if the shame isn't going to keep up its end of the bargain?

Kai: This isn't where I thought we'd be going with this. This is weird.

Psychiatrist: Shame is a weird creature. The very things you do to control shame, to keep it out of your face, are the very same things that make shame grow. You check out of everything that matters to you in order to avoid feeling shame. And when you disappear from the areas of life that are most important to you, you build in another layer of self-blame— and then you feel even more shame.

Kai: I get what you're saying, but I don't know what to do. I'm lost and I feel powerless. I've lost too much. I've thought a lot about killing myself over these years.

Psychiatrist: I'd be surprised if you hadn't thought about it, to be honest with you. That's another way to sit down, shut up, and disappear.

Kai: That's a depressing way to think about it. If I stay around, shame gets the upper hand. If I kill myself, shame gets the upper hand.

Psychiatrist: Only if you follow the pact you've made with shame to keep it under wraps.

Kai: What are you saying? That I can just walk away from my shame? Just forget about all that I've been through? All the mistakes I've made?

Psychiatrist: No, not at all. You've been through what you've been through. That's going to be in your memory banks until the day you die. What I'm curious about is what would happen if you *stopped* agreeing to sit down, shut up, and disappear?

Kai: Even if I wanted to do that, I don't know what else to do.

Psychiatrist: The opposite of sitting down is to stand up—for what you hold important. The opposite of shutting up is to speak out. And the opposite of disappearing from your life is to reappear. Can you think of some small ways that you could do any one of those three things?

Kai: Wow! The thought of doing any of that makes me shaky inside. Very scary! I guess I've gotten used to not having a life, as weird as that sounds.

Psychiatrist: Human beings can get used to almost any kind of living conditions. So, sure, this stuff is definitely not the norm for you right now, and doing anything like standing up for what you believe in, speaking your mind, or reappearing in life will seem new and awkward at first. But here is the crux: if you listen very closely, the part of you that feels shame will also rejoice if you *do* go out into the world again. Your sense of shame also reflects your deepest values, what you hold important, what you're seeking in your life. Only, its message is coming in a backhanded way, and the only way to get from where you are to where you want to be is to go after what matters to you.

Kai: (*long pause*) So, standing up, speaking out…. What was the third thing?

Psychiatrist: Reappearing.

Kai: The thing is, where do I start?

Psychiatrist: It doesn't matter. Any little thing will do. It's all best done in baby steps.

Kai: Okay, baby steps.

Psychiatrist: Any small change in tactics is a great place to begin. Can you think of anything?

Kai: I could begin with Jim, I guess. We were really tight, and I just blew him off. I feel really shitty about that. He tried to reach out to me several times, wanted to get together and have lunch, but I always came up with an excuse. I think he just kinda gave up on trying to help me or be my friend. He has a big presence on social media—he's an IT guy—and every once in a while I go online and read his posts.

> Psychiatrist: So, what would standing up for what you care about look like with Jim? What would speaking out look like? What would reappearing look like?
>
> Kai: I guess, like suggesting we get together or something like that. But to do that seems a big deal to me.
>
> Psychiatrist: You're absolutely free to set the dial anywhere you want. What could you do that for you would represent being a friend to Jim? Whatever you pick should be something that, for you, is important in a friendship. Jim may have moved on in his life, you know that, so this is more about you and what you want to stand for. He may or may not be interested; we don't know what will happen. But you can come out to the edge of your comfort zone and do what you believe in. This is what it means to check back into your life. Little actions that reflect what you believe in.
>
> Kai: I think sending him a message will do. Okay. Maybe I'll tell him that I'd like to get together for lunch sometime and that I'll understand if he doesn't want to do that.
>
> Psychiatrist: That is very, very cool. Right from the heart.
>
> Kai: (*Looks down.*) Yeah. I got lots of rebuilding to do.
>
> Psychiatrist: And new building to do. On a scale of 1 to 10, where 1 is you're not confident at all you will actually contact Jim, and 10 means you're completely confident you will, where would you put yourself?
>
> Kai: I would say 8 or 9. I know that I'll be anxious about it, but it's the right thing to do to clear the air with him.

In the use of ACT with patients in chronic states of crisis, patience and persistence are two of the psychiatrist's most important virtues. As Kai's case demonstrates, one obviously cannot change the entirety of a patient's life in a single consultation. It is more realistic to see the meeting as offering some seeds, planting them, watering them, and then seeing if any of the seeds germinate and grow. Some will, some won't, but the beauty of ACT is the life-changing effect when any seedling takes hold.

In this session, the psychiatrist started by probing for values. This immediately brought Kai's deep sense of shame into the picture. The focus shifted to helping Kai stay present to this very uncomfortable feeling, a skill that might help him refrain from either sinking into his dark world of loss, self-rejection, and isolation or seeking to avoid distress. The psychiatrist's suggestion that he be curious about and stay present to the feeling of shame led to a moment of mindfulness. In Figure 4–1, mindfulness was one level up (Level 3) from entanglement and identification with experience (Level 2), on one hand, and suppression and avoidance of experience (also Level 2), on the other. Mindfully, we notice the ubiquitous desire and aversion; we witness the ancient impulses to grip and to push away experience.

Patients are often told to try not to avoid anxiety or other feelings—words to the effect of "avoid avoiding." But it is not easy to perform such a negation of a negation. It's more helpful to offer patients another way of relating to their agony and understanding their avoidance behavior. By explicitly welcoming Kai's shame into the room, the psychiatrist acknowledged that the experience of shame is allowed and can be accepted for what it is: a feeling. Kai doesn't have to try to eradicate it. It will be there when it is there, and it won't be there when it isn't. His best hope of changing his relationship with shame is to learn how to be "in it" as well as "with it," rather than to avoid it. The psychiatrist introduces the metaphor of a "pact" between Kai and his shame in order to help him find the observational distance he needs so he can form a new relationship with the shame. He doesn't have to live his life quietly to keep his shame at bay. He can live boldly, follow his values, and take his shame along for the ride. The aim of a conversation about values and committed actions is to get the patient to agree to try something different that reflects their needs and values. In Kai's case, given his condition of stasis in life, no behavior would be too small to consider as the next step, so long as it were true to his values.

We don't know what eventually happened in Kai's life; that is a common denouement of one-time crisis consultations. But we do know that he acquired a powerful tool with which to explore what is important to him. The psychiatrist focused on helping Kai connect with his values, clouded though they were by his comprehensive efforts to control his sense of shame; the consultation did not directly jump to decision-making or cognitive problem-solving. When Kai ends his pact with shame, which, together with avoidance of fear, has organized his life for 7 years, he will ask himself, "Now that my life is no longer organized around controlling my sense of fear and shame, what *will* it be organized around?" The answer, hopefully, is that it will become organized around his values of friendliness, authentic relating, and creativity in work, among other things. When he is connected to his values, he will be able to gauge the viability of actions he is contemplating by asking himself, "Is this action in accord with what I value most?" and "Am I doing what is important to me now?" If the answer is no, he can change course. If it's yes, he will be more inclined to keep going even in those moments when his fear and shame reappear and he has an impulse to control it.

The psychiatrist also asked Kai to be mindful of the rewarding experience inherent to values-consistent behavior, regardless of its outcome. He will be acting in line with his value of nourishing his friendships when he contacts Jim, even if Jim is no longer interested in being Kai's friend. The latter is certainly a possibility but is not a reason for Kai to avoid acting, at last, according to his value of showing up for people he cares about. Reminding himself of his values while he acts on them will allow him to fully know, feel, and benefit from the gratifying quality of engagement.

We are not talking about the short-term reward that can be had from acting in accordance with one's desire to have one more ice cream or to play one more computer game. There is nothing wrong with enjoying an ice cream or a computer game. Indeed, there is nothing morally reprehensible in grasping short-term pleasures or avoiding discomfort. But we have everything to gain if we stay connected to and act in consonance with our long-term values. Kai will not succeed in his quest to reclaim his life from his pact with shame if he remains too focused on immediate rewards or punishments. If we pay attention, we notice that the ice cream type of reward is over when it is over, whereas the rewarding experience of acting in accordance with long-term values becomes enriched over time. Values such as equanimity, clarity, kindness, compassion, play, and purpose are infinite and timeless by nature. The more we connect to them, express them, act true to them, give space to them, and embody them, the more they enrich our life. Values cannot be consumed, they do not run out, and they are not achieved and left behind. They remain an unfinished journey of discovery until the day of our demise.

Patience and Persistence in Crisis Integration

Although each of us tends to feel alone in our suffering, and sometimes we blame ourselves for it, the processes that lead to crisis instigation are neither personal nor unique. They originate in the ways that we human beings have learned about the world and our place in it: in the way the brain makes predictions based on the past; the way we learn how to avoid threats and to approach opportunities; the way the brain generates a sense of self; the way we learn to behave to obtain safety, approval, and care within a social group as we grow up; and the way that language enables previously learned rules to govern our behavior. Internally, these ways of learning lead to both an overidentification with and an avoidance of inner affliction as well as an attachment to strategies that have helped us to reduce emotional pain in the past. These propensities may well have helped us to survive and protected us from certain kinds of pain and discomfort, but they don't provide the kind of flexibility needed in a crisis.

In this book, we have suggested that a crisis is instigated when something adverse happens to us; we then try to avoid feeling the emotions and bodily sensations that naturally arise in response to that adverse event and, at the same time, disengage by clinging to behavioral strategies that have ceased to be useful. The persistent use of avoidant coping is not a benign process; it will become a major driver of disengagement from life. Neither is disengagement a benign process, for it will trigger a second wave of distressing emotions in reaction to a mounting list of needs whose fulfillment is deeply desired but that remain unmet.

Fortunately, the human brain gives us an inherent ability to observe and evaluate the utility of previous learning. We can contemplate the behavioral strategies we are using and the verbal rules that are guiding us. We can become aware of our feelings, bodily sensations, met and unmet needs, and deeply held values. This witnessing capacity provides the basis for the new learning and the psychological flexibility required to integrate a crisis.

The practice of not getting lost in inner experiences—neither reacting to them nor trying to get rid of them, argue with them, or judge them—is for many people a new way of relating to their inner life. The capacity to merely observe everything that is going on inside us is, paradoxically, both simple and intricate. In clinical practice, therefore, the introduction of this witnessing perspective is an exercise in direct experience rather than a matter of intellectual argument. The psychiatrist can both model calm witnessing of the turmoil of crisis and give patients moment-to-moment coaching in how to go about experiencing this themselves.

We've suggested that the psychiatrist teach the use of neutral internal bodily sensations to provide an attentional anchor. When emotions are intense, neutral bodily areas are commonly ones outside the torso, such as the feet or hands, but there are good alternatives to which the patient's attention may first be directed, such as sounds or the silence between sounds. Any of these techniques will help the patient to slow down, unify their attention, and witness their pain from an ever less perturbable state of being. When outer holding is unavailable or insufficient, which is often the case for patients in crisis, this mindful outlook will help provide the necessary holding and create conditions under which the somatic distress and emotional pain of the situation will gradually settle down. This process is gradual partly because some degree of bias—wanting less or more of a certain type of inner experience—will, in the heat of crisis, sneak into the picture and color the witnessing perspective. Mindfulness is thus an iterative process in which we become increasingly aware and accepting of all the ways we cling to strategies that help us avoid emotional pain, as well as accepting of the pain itself. If we remain observant, we will with time gain more and more nuance of perception and wisdom about what is actually happening. For example, because present-moment experience builds on past experiences, mindfulness of what is going on in the present also means being mindful of what has come before.

If new learning is to be gained about unhelpful prior knowledge, compassion must be involved. When we are criticized or judged, whether by others or ourselves, we can become too scared to let go of old unworkable strategies. Thus, it is helpful to bring into play our inherent capacity to extend care and kindness to ourselves and others. When held lightly and tenderly, both our painful inner experiences and our sense of a criticized self become less burdensome and less opaque and thus easier to accept.

Although everyone has the potential to exercise mindfulness, acceptance, compassion, and engagement, in the context of a crisis these abilities need to be cultivated and practiced. Indeed, we can make the most of the motivation to seek new forms of learning that can arise in a crisis. The extent to which we manage to exercise these integrative processes in each moment will build upon the extent to which we've done so in previous moments. They are like muscles that need to be used in order to gain and retain strength. Unlike muscular power, however, these capacities are boundless. There is no limit to how much presence, peace, kindness, and care we can offer ourselves and bring into the world.

Just as avoidance and disengagement are the core processes of crisis instigation, acceptance and engagement are central to crisis integration, and both are mediated by mindfulness. They equate to mindful being and mindful doing. Acceptance and engagement are more intertwined in crisis integration than it may at first seem. Each tends to elicit the other. Acceptance of our inner and outer predicaments will bring the clarity needed to engage wisely with the world. In a crisis, feelings speak loudly of the patient's unmet needs and values. When they mindfully and compassionately embrace their feelings, they can stay in the moment and learn what truly matters to them—what they wish for themselves and for others. Getting to know their values will prove to be both essential and fruitful because one's values provide the most useful guide for one's actions in a challenging situation. Meanwhile, engagement will expand their willingness to make contact with both the devastating emotions of the crisis situation and any additional discomfort that arises when they act in accordance with personal values in ways counter to previous learning.

In times of personal crisis, we are sorely tempted to believe that there must be something better than just opening up to the pain of the moment while engaging with the world according to our values. Surely there must be some other option? Something that offers a quicker remedy? Unfortunately, all of the quick remedies share one common feature: they work for a while, and then they make things worse. They don't end the pain; they amplify it. There really isn't any better pathway through than to bring a compassionate gaze to what is here.

Our hope is that readers will find this book to be a source of inspiration they will return to again and again. The kind of learning it elucidates is gradual. We encourage psychiatrists to try out different ways of supporting patients' acceptance and engagement processes, because patients' histories and circumstances will vary greatly. Clinical interventions should be tailored to fit not only the patient's specific learning style and present predicament but also the psychiatrist's personal teaching style. We invite you, the reader, to be gentle with yourself. Just as we psychiatrists aim to be patient and supportive with someone in crisis, we ought not expect ourselves to be perfect when we're trying out new things.

Everyone goes through times when we feel like the rug has been pulled out from under us, when what we have trusted and loved is lost, changed, or endangered. As much as we would like to save others and ourselves from such afflictions, the heartbreaking truth is that we cannot always prevent them. They are part of the human condition. The task for anyone who has suffered in such a way is to learn how to be with the hardship in a way that most enhances their life, and to serve others while they do the same. Crises bear upon existential matters, so this obliges us to go deep to the core of what it means to be human. However, it is not only about going deep; it is also about *how* we do so.

Crisis integration requires gentleness and forbearance. Certainly, people sometimes have an epiphany that changes them altogether in one go, but that is rare. If all the answers were readily available to us, we would not be in a crisis in the first place. Most of us need to learn our lessons in our own time. We avoid, we cling, we identify with experiences, we act according to previously learned and outdated rules, we create more trouble, and we suffer. Then there are moments when we're able to let go of avoiding and clinging and instead mindfully face our inner pain, explore our needs and values, and try out new valued and useful actions. Our task in a crisis is to gracefully accept the whole experience—to notice "Oh no, here I go again" and then to tell ourselves, "This too is okay." It is comforting to know that, although the moments when we're able to be truly present to what's going on and to do something new may seem few, those fleeting moments do cumulatively add up to produce healing and positive change.

References

Aknin LB, Hamlin JK, Dunn EW: Giving leads to happiness in young children. PLoS One 7(6):e39211, 2012 22720078

Aknin LB, Dunn EW, Proulx J, et al: Does spending money on others promote happiness? A registered replication report. J Pers Soc Psychol 119(2):e15–e26, 2020 ꞓꞵꞵꞵꝋꞵꝪꝪ

Alim TN, Feder A, Graves RE, et al: Trauma, resilience, and recovery in a high-risk African-American population. Am J Psychiatry 165(12):1566–1575, 2008 19015233

Alter C, Haynes S, Worland J: Time 2019 person of the year Greta Thunberg. Time magazine, December 11, 2019. Available at: https://www.time.com/person-of-the-year-2019-greta-thunberg/. Accessed May 16, 2022.

Barney JL, Lillis J, Haynos AF, et al: Assessing the valuing process in acceptance and commitment therapy: experts' review of the current status and recommendations for future measure development. J Contextual Behav Sci 12:225–233, 2019 31828006

Cohen S: The role of individual responsibility in the transition to environmental sustainability. State of the Planet, May 10, 2021. Available at: https://news.climate.columbia.edu/2021/05/10/the-role-of-individual-responsibility-in-the-transition-to-environmental-sustainability. Accessed May 16, 2022.

Collins AGE, Cockburn J: Beyond dichotomies in reinforcement learning. Nat Rev Neurosci 21(10):576–586, 2020 32873936

Cutler J, Wittmann MK, Abdurahman A, et al: Ageing is associated with disrupted reinforcement learning whilst learning to help others is preserved. Nat Commun 12(1):4440, 2021 34290236

Duckworth A: Grit: Why Passion and Resilience are the Secrets to Success. London, Ebury Publishing, 2017

Dunn EW, Aknin LB, Norton MI: Prosocial spending and happiness. Curr Dir Psychol Sci 23:41–47, 2014

Feder A, Mota N, Salim R, et al: Risk, coping and PTSD symptom trajectories in World Trade Center responders. J Psychiatr Res 82:68–79, 2016 27468166

Fehr E, Fischbacher U: The nature of human altruism. Nature 425(6960):785–791, 2003 14574401

FeldmanHall O, Dalgleish T, Evans D, et al: Empathic concern drives costly altruism. Neuroimage 105:347–356, 2015 25462694

Hailes HP, Yu R, Danese A, et al: Long-term outcomes of childhood sexual abuse: an umbrella review. Lancet Psychiatry 6(10):830–839, 2019 31519507

Harbaugh WT, Mayr U, Burghart DR: Neural responses to taxation and voluntary giving reveal motives for charitable donations. Science 316(5831):1622–1625, 2007 17569866

Iigaya K, Hauser TU, Kurth-Nelson Z, et al: The value of what's to come: neural mechanisms coupling prediction error and the utility of anticipation. Sci Adv 6(25):eaba3828, 2020 32596456

Isaacs K, Mota NP, Tsai J, et al: Psychological resilience in U.S. military veterans: a 2-year, nationally representative prospective cohort study. J Psychiatr Res 84:301–309, 2017 27814502

Levermann A: Individuals can't solve the climate crisis: governments need to step up. The Guardian, July 10, 2019. Available at: https://www.theguardian.com/

commentisfree/2019/jul/10/individuals-climate-crisis-government-planet-priority. Accessed May 16, 2022.

Nasser HM, Calu DJ, Schoenbaum G, et al: The dopamine prediction error: contributions to associative models of reward learning. Front Psychol 8:244, 2017 28275359

Nezu AM, Nezu CM, D'Zurilla T: Problem-Solving Therapy: A Treatment Manual. New York, Springer, 2013

Park CL: Making sense of the meaning literature: an integrative review of meaning making and its effects on adjustment to stressful life events. Psychol Bull 136(2):257–301, 2010 20192563

Piech RM, Strelchuk D, Knights J, et al: People with higher interoceptive sensitivity are more altruistic, but improving interoception does not increase altruism. Sci Rep 7:15652, 2017

Rigitano E: COP24, the speech by 15-year-old climate activist Greta Thunberg everyone should listen to. Lifegate, December 17, 2018. Available at: https://www.lifegate.com/greta-thunberg-speech-cop24. Accessed May 16, 2022.

Schaefer SM, Morozink Boylan J, van Reekum CM, et al: Purpose in life predicts better emotional recovery from negative stimuli. PLoS One 8(11):e80329, 2013 24236176

Schultz W: Dopamine neurons and their role in reward mechanisms. Curr Opin Neurobiol 7(2):191–197, 1997 9142754

Southwick SM, Charney DS: Resilience: The Science of Mastering Life's Greatest Challenges. Cambridge, UK, Cambridge University Press, 2012

Thunberg G: "I want you to panic": 16-year-old issues climate warning at Davos. The Guardian, January 25, 2019. Available at: https://www.theguardian.com/science/video/2019/jan/25/i-want-you-to-panic-16-year-old-greta-thunberg-issues-climate-warning-at-davos-video. Accessed May 16, 2022.

Tsai J, El-Gabalawy R, Sledge WH, et al: Post-traumatic growth among veterans in the USA: results from the National Health and Resilience in Veterans Study. Psychol Med 45(1):165–179, 2015 25065450

Voon V, Reiter A, Sebold M, et al: Model-based control in dimensional psychiatry. Biol Psychiatry 82(6):391–400, 2017 28599832

Wang Y, Ge J, Zhang H, et al: Altruistic behaviors relieve physical pain. Proc Natl Acad Sci USA 117(2):950–958, 2020 31888986

Zaki J, Mitchell JP: Equitable decision making is associated with neural markers of intrinsic value. Proc Natl Acad Sci USA 108(49):19761–19766, 2011 22106300

Index

*Page numbers printed in **boldface** type refer to figures.*

functions of immediate
consequences and, 201
vs. goals, 201
vs. rules and strategies, 200

Vulnerability, factors linked to mental
health, 16, **17**
World Health Organization (WHO), 20